Norbert Rietbrock
Barry G. Woodcock
A. Horst Staib
Dieter Loew

Drug Absorption at Different Regions of the Human Gastro-Intestinal Tract: Methods of Investigation and Results

Arzneimittelabsorption aus verschiedenen Bereichen des Gastrointestinaltraktes beim Menschen: Untersuchungsmethoden und Ergebnisse

N. Rietbrock and B.G. Woodcock (Eds.)

Methods in Clinical Pharmacology

Proceedings Series of the Annual International Symposia held in Frankfurt

Number 1
Methods in Clinical Pharmacology,
co-edited by G. Neuhaus. 1980

Number 2
Progress in Protein Binding,
volume assisted by A. Laßmann. 1981

Number 3
Theophylline and other Methylxanthines,
co-edited by A.H. Staib. 1982

Number 4
Color Vision in Clinical Pharmacology. 1983

Number 5
Balanced Alpha/Beta Blockade of Adrenoceptors.
A Rational Therapeutic Concept in the Treatment
of Hypertension and Coronary Heart Disease. 1984

Number 6
Clinical Pharmacology in the Aged. 1985

Number 7
**Drug Absorption at Different Regions of the
Human Gastro-Intestinal Tract:
Methods of Investigation and Results,**
co-edited by A.H. Staib and D. Loew. 1987

Norbert Rietbrock, Barry G. Woodcock, A. Horst Staib,
Dieter Loew (Editors)

Methods in Clinical Pharmacology
Number 7

Drug Absorption at Different Regions of the Human Gastro-Intestinal Tract: Methods of Investigation and Results

Proceedings of an International Workshop on
Methods in Clinical Pharmacology Frankfurt, November 14, 1986

Arzneimittelabsorption aus verschiedenen Bereichen des Gastrointestinaltraktes beim Menschen: Untersuchungsmethoden und Ergebnisse

Vorträge und Diskussionen auf einem Internationalen
Workshop „Methods in Clinical Pharmacology"
Frankfurt, 14. November 1986

V Friedr. Vieweg & Sohn
Braunschweig / Wiesbaden

The Editors

Norbert Rietbrock is Professor and Head of the Department of Clinical Pharmacology, University Clinic, Frankfurt am Main, FRG.

Barry G. Woodcock is Senior Lecturer in Clinical Pharmacology, University Clinic, Frankfurt am Main, FRG.

A. Horst Staib is Professor of Clinical Pharmacology, University Clinic, Frankfurt am Main, FRG.

Dieter Loew is Head of Clinical Research, MEDICE Pharmaceuticals, Iserlohn and Wuppertal, FRG.

Vieweg is a subsidiary company of the Bertelsmann Publishing Group.

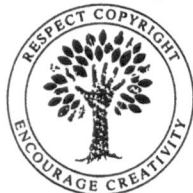
Set by Frohberg, Freigericht
Produced by Lengericher Handelsdruckerei, Lengerich

ISBN 978-3-528-07944-4   ISBN 978-3-322-91091-2 (eBook)
DOI 10.1007/978-3-322-91091-2

Contents / Inhaltsverzeichnis

VI

„Unter Resorption eines chemischen Agens verstehen wir seine Aufnahme aus dem Milieu exterieur oder aus örtlich begrenzten Stellen des Körperinneren in die Lymph- und Blutbahn."

Werner Scheler 1980

"Absorption may be described as the rate at which a drug leaves its site of administration and the extent to which this occurs."

Goodman and Gilman 1985

Program of the Workshop

November 14, 1986;
14.00–18.00 hours

Chairman:
Prof. Dr. N. Rietbrock

Prof. Dr. A.H. Staib
Priv.-Doz. Dr. Dr. D. Loew
Dr. B.G. Woodcock

N. Rietbrock, (Frankfurt):
Eröffnung und Themeneinführung

J. Hirtz, (Paris):
The use of intubation techniques to study drug
absorption in humans

Diskussion: *Drewe (Basel):*
Untersuchung des Absorptionsverhaltens mittels
einer zweilumigen Sondentechnik

J. Ulmius, et al. (Lund):
Simultaneous pharmacokinetic and in vivo
gamma scintigraphic monitoring as an aid in the
development of an enprofylline SR-tablet

J. Caldwell, et al. (London):
Stable isotopes for in vivo studies of SR-prepara-
tions

O. Schuster, B. Hugemann, (Frankfurt):
Entwicklungsweg der HF-Kapsel, Varianten
und methodentypische Befunde

K.-H. Antonin, P. Bieck, (Tübingen):
Coloskopische und Stoma-Methoden zur Untersuchung der enteralen Arzneimittel-Absorption

Round-Table:
angemeldete Diskussionsbeiträge

R. Joeres, G. Hofstetter, E. Richter (Würzburg):
Coffein- und Hexobarbitalresorption bei Patienten mit Lebercirrhose und portaler Hypertension

S. Hotchkiss, J. Caldwell, (London):
Influence of absorption rate on the metabolic
kinetics of theophylline

H. Oelschläger, D. Rotley, (Frankfurt):
Metabolisierung von Fosfestrol durch die
Darmschleimhaut

A.H. Staib, et al. (Frankfurt):
Theophyllin-Absorption in verschiedenen
Darmabschnitten

Diskussion: *Lippold (Düsseldorf):*
Hinweise über die Resorption von Theophyllin
aus dem Dickdarm nach einer Depotarzneiform

Hellenbrecht, Frankfurt:
Retardierungsprobleme bei Theophyllin-
Präparaten

D. Loew, et al. (Frankfurt/Iserlohn):
Lokalisation der Absorption von Furosemid:
Befunde und Folgerungen für verschiedene Dar-
reichungsformen

H. Laufen, A. Wildfeuer, (Illertissen):
Resorption von Isosorbid-5-Mononitrat aus
dem Gastrointestinaltrakt

D. Brockmeier, H.-G. Grigoleit (Frankfurt):
Gastro-Intestinale Arzneimittelabsorption:
Physikochemische und biomathematische As-
pekte

B.G. Woodcock, (Frankfurt):
Effect of dissolution rate on verapamil absorption

D. Brachtel, E. Richter, (Würzburg):
Coffeinresorption bei veränderter Magenent-
leerung

A.H. Staib, (Frankfurt):
Schlußwort

VIII

Adressen der Autoren

Dr. K.-H. Antonin
Humanpharmakologisches Institut
Ciba-Geigy GmbH
Ob dem Himmelreich 7
D-7400 Tübingen

Prof. Dr. P. Bieck
Humanpharmakologisches Institut
Ciba-Geigy GmbH
Ob dem Himmelreich 7
D-7400 Tübingen

Dr. O. Borga
AB Draco
Box 34
S-22100 Lund

PD Dr. Brachtel
Krankenanstalt Mutterhaus
der Borromäerinnen
Medizinische Abteilung
Feldstraße 16, Postfach 2920
D-5500 Trier

Dr. D. Brockmeier
Klinische Forschung, Abt. Biometrie
Hoechst AG
Postfach 800320
D-6230 Frankfurt/Main 80

Dr. J. Caldwell
St. Mary's Hospital Medical School
Department of Pharmacology and Toxicology
London W21PG
U.K.

A. Fischer
Abt. Klinische Pharmakologie
Klinikum der J.W. Goethe-Universität
Theodor-Stern-Kai 7
D-6000 Frankfurt/Main 70

Prof. Dr. Dr. E.H. Graul
Institut für Environtologie und Nuklearmedizin
Philipps-Universität Marburg
und MEDICEF-Institute, Miami/USA
Bahnhofstraße 7
D-3550 Marburg

Dr. H.-G. Grigoleit
Verkauf Pharma, Zentrales Marketing
Hoechst AG
Postfach 800320
D-6230 Frankfurt/Main 80

Dr. S. Harder
Abt. Klinische Pharmakologie
Klinikum der J.W. Goethe-Universität
Theodor-Stern-Kai 7
D-6000 Frankfurt/Main 70

PD Dr. D. Hellenbrecht
Zentrum der Pharmakologie
Klinikum der J.W. Goethe-Universität
Theodor-Stern-Kai 7
D-6000 Frankfurt/Main 70

Dr. C.-D. Herzfeldt
Institut für Pharmazeutische Technologie
J.W. Goethe-Universität
Georg-Voigt-Straße 16
D-6000 Frankfurt/Main 11

Dr. J. Hirtz
Biopharmaceutical Evaluation Company
B.P.67.
F-92152 Suresnes Cedex

Dr. G. Hofstetter
Medizinische Universitäts-Klinik Würzburg
Josef-Schneider-Straße 2
D-8700 Würzburg

Dr. Sharon Hotchkiss
St. Mary's Hospital Medical School
Department of Pharmacology and Toxicology
London W21PG
U.K.

Ing. B. Hugemann
Heinrich-Seliger-Straße 49
D-6000 Frankfurt/Main 71

Dr. R. Joeres
Medizinische Universitätsklinik Würzburg
Josef-Schneider-Straße 2
D-8700 Würzburg

Dr. H. Klinker
Medizinische Universitäts-Klinik Würzburg
Josef-Schneider-Straße 2
D-8700 Würzburg

Dr. H. Köhne
Dept. Analytical Development
Dr. Rentschler Arzneimittel GmbH & Co.
Mittelstraße 18
D-7958 Laupheim

Prof. Dr. J. Kollath
Zentrum der Radiologie
Klinikum der J.W. Goethe-Universität
Theodor-Stern-Kai 7
D-6000 Frankfurt/Main 70

Dr. H. Laufen
Heinrich Mack Nachf.
Abt. Pharmakologie
D-7918 Illertissen

Prof. Dr. B. C. Lippold
Institut für Pharmazeutische Technologie
Universität Düsseldorf
Universitätsstraße 1
D-4000 Düsseldorf 1

PD Dr. Dr. D. Loew
Medice Pharmazeutische Fabrik
Postfach 2063
D-5860 Iserlohn

Dr. G. Menke
Abt. Klinische Pharmakologie
Klinikum der J.W. Goethe-Universität
Theodor-Stern-Kai 7
D-6000 Frankfurt/Main 70

Prof. Dr. H. Oelschläger
Institut für Pharmazeutische Chemie
J.W. Goethe-Universität
Georg-Voigt-Straße 14
D-6000 Frankfurt/Main

Prof. Dr. E. Richter
Medizinische Universitäts-Klinik Würzburg
Josef-Schneider-Straße 2
D-8700 Würzburg

Prof. Dr. N. Rietbrock
Abt. Klinische Pharmakologie
Klinikum der J.W. Goethe-Universität
Theodor-Stern-Kai 7
D-6000 Frankfurt/Main 70

Dr. D. Rothley
Institut für Pharmazeutische Chemie
J.W. Goethe-Universität Frankfurt
Georg-Voigt-Straße 14
D-6000 Frankfurt/Main

Dr. O. Schuster
PAZ GmbH
In der Schildwacht 13
D-6230 Frankfurt/Main 80

Prof. Dr. A. H. Staib
Abt. Klinische Pharmakologie
Klinikum der J.W. Goethe-Universität
Theodor-Stern-Kai 7
D-6000 Frankfurt/Main 70

Dr. J. Ulmius
AB Draco
Box 34
S-22100 Lund

Dr. Z.G. Wagner
Fyzikon AB
Box 120
S-22100 Lund

Prof. Dr. A. Wildfeuer
Direktion Forschung und Entwicklung
Heinrich Mack Nachf.
D-7918 Illertissen

Dr. P. Wollmer
Dept. Clinical Physiology
University of Lund
S-22100 Lund

Dr. B.G. Woodcock
Abt. Klinische Pharmakologie,
Klinikum der J.W. Goethe-Universität
Theodor-Stern-Kai 7
D-6000 Frankfurt/Main 70

Prof. Dr. W. Zilly
Hartwald-Klinik der BfA
Schlüchterner Straße 4
D-8788 Bad Brückenau

Eröffnung und Themeneinführung

N. Rietbrock

Wachsendes Qualitätsbewußtsein beschränkt sich nicht nur auf die Güter des täglichen Bedarfs, sondern gilt auch für die im Krankheitsfall zu verordnenden Arzneimittel. Die Qualität ist vom pharmazeutischen Hersteller im Zulassungsverfahren nachzuweisen. So schreibt der im zweiten Gesetz zur Änderung des Arzneimittelgesetzes vom 16. August 1986 neu eingefügte § 11a bindend vor, daß in der Fachinformation „die pharmakologischen und toxikologischen Eigenschaften und Angaben über die Pharmakokinetik und Bioverfügbarkeit, soweit diese Angaben für die therapeutische Anwendung erforderlich sind . . ." enthalten sein müssen.

Damit schränkt der Gesetzgeber aber auch bewußt die Angaben zur Pharmakokinetik und Bioverfügbarkeit auf therapeutisch relevante Arzneigruppen ein. Folglich bleibt die Erbringung der Daten praktikabel. Es liegt nicht im Sinne des Gesetzgebers noch in dem des Herstellers in Anbetracht der limitierten Zahl der medizinischen Institute mit entsprechender Ausrichtung, des relativ großen Zeitaufwandes und der nicht unerheblichen Kosten für alle Arzneimittel eine generelle Regelung zu treffen.

Pharmakokinetik und Bioverfügbarkeit sind für die therapeutische Anwendung erforderlich unter anderem

bei Arzneimitteln, die bei Überdosierungen zu gravierenden unerwünschten Wirkungen führen können;

bei Arzneimitteln, die vorwiegend renal eliminiert werden und bei denen die Gefahr einer verstärkten Kumulation bei eingeschränkter Nierenfunktion besteht;

bei Arzneimitteln mit einem „first pass" Effekt;

bei allen Arzneimitteln mit geringer therapeutischer Breite.

Damit wird aber auch der Zweck solcher Studien klar: Qualität ist ein relatives Merkmal eines Arzneimittels. Die Validität dieses Merkmals ist immer im Zusammenhang mit dem klinischen Krankheitsbild zu sehen.

Bioverfügbarkeitsstudien haben nun einen materiell-inhaltlichen und einen methodischen Sektor. Der materiell-inhaltliche Sektor kann nur von dem physiologisch und pathophysiologisch geschulten Arzt beurteilt werden. Im Vorfeld dieser Beurteilung liegt der methodische Sektor, in dem Verfahrensweisen entsprechend der wissenschaftlichen und technischen Weiterentwicklung dem jeweiligen Erkenntnisstand anzupassen sind. Ferner darf bei Beschreibung und Beurteilung der Bioverfügbarkeit nicht ein pharmakokinetischer und statistischer Schematismus um sich greifen. Es ist weder wünschenswert noch sinnvoll, detaillierte Kriterien für jeden nur denkbaren Einzelfall generell von vornherein festlegen zu wollen. Dies dient nicht dem Zweck eines auf Wirksamkeit und Sicherheit gerichteten Arzneimittelgesetzes.

Es gilt in erster Linie mit geeigneten Methoden die funktionellen Vorgänge bei der Resorption zu hinterfragen. Dieses war das Anliegen von Prof. Staib, Dr. Loew, Dr. Woodcock und von mir bei der Zusammenstellung der Vorträge. Dabei gingen wir von dem

Konzept aus, daß für die klinisch-therapeutische Bewertung der Resorptionsphänomene beim Menschen zunächst die Frage nach der Spezifität und Kapazität der Transportvorgänge und ihre Verteilung auf die einzelnen Darmabschnitte von Bedeutung ist. Diese Frage bedarf beim Menschen noch der eingehenden Untersuchung. Erfolgsversprechende Ansätze dazu sollen heute diskutiert werden.

Ich danke Ihnen, daß Sie unserer Einladung gefolgt sind.

Intubation Techniques for the Study of the Absorption of Drugs in Man

J. Hirtz
Ciba-Geigy Pharmaceutical Development, CH-4002 Basle,
Biopharmaceutical Evaluation Company, B.P.67, F-92152 Suresnes Cedex

Summary

Intubation techniques have been used for several decades to investigate digestive processes in man. They became quantitative when non-absorbable markers were introduced. Later on multichannel tubes made it possible to perform simultaneous measurements at different levels in the gastrointestinal tract. We are using them since 1981 to explore the absorption of drugs from the stomach to the colon. Different variants of the method have been necessary to explore the different levels of the gastrointestinal tract.

Gastric, duodenal and upper jejunal absorptions were determined simultaneously. A tube was placed in the stomach and three others in the small intestine: one at the level of the papilla, the second at the angle of Treitz and the third 30 cm further down. The studied drug (metoprolol) was introduced in the empty stomach with a liquid meal containing ^{14}C-PEG 4000. A solution of unlabelled PEG 4000 was perfused at a constant rate below the pylorus. Luminal samples were collected at intervals in the stomach, at the end of the duodenum and in the jejunum.

To investigate ileal absorption, a multichannel tube with an inflatable balloon was used which prevented digestive secretions reaching the studied segment. One non-absorbable marker was added to the drug solution in saline. Absorption rates in the ileum were compared to those in the jejunum in the same subjects on two different days by allowing the tube to spontaneously move from jejunum to ileum.

Colonic absorption could not be studied directly. A simple comparison between the plasma profiles obtained in the same subjects when a drug solution was infused at a constant rate either in the jejunum or in the colon was performed.

These investigations demonstrated that metoprolol is absorbed at similar rates all along the gastrointestinal tract. In addition these investigations revealed that food, but not digestive secretions, increases the absorption rate. They provided interesting findings about the physiological effects of metoprolol. These studies demonstrated the validity of the intubation techniques to investigate drug absorption in humans. Nevertheless, they are extremely time consuming and require the collaboration of well trained gastroenterologists.

Most drugs are given orally, but little is known about their absorption in the gastrointestinal (GI) tract of man [1]. The largest part of the presently available information has been obtained indirectly, by using a pharmacokinetic treatment of plasma concentration-time profiles. When a drug can be administered to the same subjects intravenously and orally, it is possible to build up a model simulating the absorption profile [2]. Even if the intravenous administration is not permitted, special pharmacokinetic techniques allow such a model to be obtained [3, 4]. Nevertheless, the indirect pharmacokinetic approach generally considers the absorption process as a whole, and it is unable to estimate the absorption rate at the various absorption sites of the GI tract.

The only way to obtain a complete and detailed picture of the absorption processes in man is to measure the disappearance of the drug from the various parts of the GI tract. This procedure has been used for a long time to study the absorption and digestion of nutrients, it has been progressively sophisticated and validated, and it is surprising that it has not yet been used to investigate the absorption of drugs, except on rare occasions.

This paper will describe some variants of this technique as far as they can be applied to the problem of drug absorption in man, and give an example of the results they can provide.

The first studies on the physiology of digestion were based on a balance method, i.e. the comparison of the amount ingested and that recovered from the GI tract. A simple tube was used to collect the luminal fluid, but this did not permit precise measurements as only a fraction of the fluid passing at the sampling site was collected. In 1936, Abbott and Miller [5] proposed an improved procedure: a segment of the intestine was isolated between two inflatable balloons, so that the whole luminal content could be collected without dilution by the digestive secretions coming from the upper part of the GI tract. But this procedure was likely to disturb the intestinal motility and the blood supply to the mucosa. Hyden in 1956 [6] demonstrated that PEG 4000 is practically not absorbed in the intestine of man, and since this time it has been widely used as a non-absorbable marker in intubation studies. As early as 1957, Borgström et al. [7] studied the intestinal digestion and absorption of a liquid meal given with PEG 4000. In 1961, Schedl and Clifton [8], and Fordtran et al. [9] proposed simultaneously the intestinal perfusion technique with markers to evaluate intraluminal water movements. This type of experiment was validated by Jacobson et al. in 1963 [10]. Later on, the intubation techniques with non-absorbable markers were extensively applied to the study of the absorption of water, electrolytes, carbohydrates, lipids, biliary salts, vitamins, etc. . . . . A more elaborate procedure was employed in 1971 by Bernier and Lebert [11] to investigate both the gastric emptying and the jejunal flow rate after the ingestion of a liquid meal. Two collection tubes were used, one in the stomach, the other in the duodenum, as well as two non-absorbable markers, one dissolved in the meal, the other perfused at a constant rate by a third tube in the duodenum, above the duodenal collection tube. This procedure was further described by Malagelada et al. [12], who applied it in extensive investigations on digestion processes.

1. The Intubation Technique

1.1 General Principles

In an intubation experiment, a solution of the drug containing a non-absorbable marker is introduced somewhere in the GI tract, and samples of the luminal fluid are collected at a definite level further down. Drug and marker concentrations are determined in the samples. As the amounts of drug and marker in the administered solution are known, and the marker is not absorbed, it is thus possible to calculate the amounts of drug remaining in each sample. The difference between the initial and the calculated amounts is assumed to correspond to the drug that has been absorbed.

It is necessary to consider here the other processes which could interfere with drug absorption and give rise to its disappearance from the GI tract. The drug could be unstable at one of the various pH encountered during its transit from the stomach to the colon. It could be metabolized by the enzymes present in the intestinal fluid, or in the mucosa. It could be degraded by the bacterial flora of the distal intestine. It could be adsorbed on the surface of the intestinal wall, or trapped inside the mucosa.

In practice, it is difficult to provide complete and unambiguous proof that the drug which disappeared from the GI tract was only absorbed and not subjected to other processes. Some separate assays may provide partial answers. The possibility of degradation at various pH can be investigated by in vitro experiments. In the same way, the incubation of the drug with freshly obtained gastric or intestinal fluids will demonstrate a metabolic degradation if any. Metabolism by intestinal tissue, or adsorption on this tissue is more difficult to study, and requires taking surgical samples. More simply, the analysis of the samples collected in the GI tract by a powerful separation technique will detect any metabolic or degradation product.

The general procedure of the technique of segmental intestinal perfusion with a non-absorbable marker is based on the following equations [13]. The part of the GI tract between the point of introduction of the drug + marker solution and the point of luminal fluid collection is called the test segment. Its length is defined by the distance between these two points, and is known from the tubes used. The rate of drug absorption in the test segment R_D is given by:

$$R_D = R_1 \cdot D_1 - R_2 \cdot D_2$$

where R_1 is the rate of infusion of the drug + marker solution, D_1 the concentration of the drug in this solution, R_2 the flow of fluid leaving the test segment and D_2 the drug concentration at the exit of the test segment. The perfusion is carried out at a known constant rate (R_1) with a solution at a known drug concentration (D_1) a fraction of which is collected at the end of the test segment, thus allowing to determine the concentration D_2. R_2 remains the only unknown data since the complete recovery of the fluid leaving the test segment is impossible. The use of the non-absorbable marker makes it possible to calculate R_2. If M_1 and M_2 are the markers concentrations at the entry and exit of the test segment:

$$R_1 M_1 = R_2 M_2$$

$$\text{and } R_2 = R_1 \frac{M_1}{M_2}$$

The rate of disappearance of the drug in the test segment R_{abs} is then given by:

$$R_{abs} = R_1D_1 - R_2D_2$$

$$= R_1D_1 - R_1 \frac{M_1}{M_2} D_2$$

$$= R_1 \left[D_1 - D_2\frac{M_1}{M_2} \right]$$

Two conditions must be fulfilled to apply this procedure:

1. a steady state exists within the test segment,
2. the luminal content in the test segment is homogenous.

The steady state condition requires that the flow rate and the drug concentration remain constant at each point of the test segment for the entire duration of the experiment. This steady state is not immediately reached, and requires a preliminary period of perfusion, which is more prolonged when the test segment is longer and/or the rate of perfusion slower. In general, a preliminary period of 30−60 minutes is sufficient to reach a steady state. However, a perfect equilibrium is never obtained due to the unavoidable variations in peristalsis and average diameter of the intestine, the irregular output of digestive secretions, and the intermittent reflux of the solution above the perfusion point. It is therefore necessary to collect a series of several samples during 10−20 minutes each to control the steady state: the marker concentration in these successive samples should not vary by more ± 10% around the mean value.

In addition, the general procedure assumes that the drug concentration in the samples collected at the end of the test segment exactly represents that of the luminal content at the sampling level, and in particular that there is no concentration gradient between the center and the periphery of the fluid column contained in the intestine. Although it is likely that the layer of fluid in contact with the mucosa undergoes more rapid exchanges with the epithelium than the fluid in the center of the lumen, pendular and peristaltic movements of the intestine, and specially circular folds, are able to achieve a good mixing of the intestinal contents. In practice, the length of the test segment is limited to 30 cm, and the reproducibility of the results obtained with a series of 6 samples showed that the homogeneity of the luminal content is satisfactory.

This general procedure is the basis of the intubation techniques used to study drug absorption. It may be applied directly to explore the upper small intestine. For the lower small intestine or the colon, as well as for the stomach, some variants of this basic technique have been developed.

1.2 Non-Absorbable Markers

Several non-absorbable markers have been employed in the past, but PEG 4000 is the most widely used. Phenolsulfonphtalein and bromosulfonphtalein are slightly absorbed in the GI tract of man, and indocyanine green seems to adhere to the mucus, at least in the dog.

PEG 4000 is neither absorbed nor destroyed in the GI tract of man. After oral administration to normal subjects, 98.2% of the dose is recovered in the feces [6]. Its solubility in water at 20°C is 62% w/w. It does not adhere to proteins and/or mucus [10]. PEG 4000 in luminal fluids may be quantitatively assayed by a turbidimetric method [14]. After elimination of the proteins by precipitation, PEG 4000 is insolubilized in a trichloroacetic acid medium, and the absorbance of the suspension is measured.

1.3 Tubes

Polyvinyl tubes with an internal diameter of 1–2 mm are used. Two or several tubes are cemented together with cyclohexanone along a segment of 20 cm. One of the tubes is radio-opaque to allow its tip to be localized fluoroscopically. At the sampling level, 10 holes are made on a length of 3 cm to facilitate the collection of the intraluminal fluid. A rubber bag containing 1 ml of mercury is attached 20 cm below the sampling site, to make the tubes move spontaneously downwards in the intestine.

The tubes are introduced through the nose of the volunteer on the evening preceding the first day of the experiment, and their position is controlled using X rays.

The experiment is started when the tube has reached the intestinal segment in which absorption is to be studied. This requires 6–12 hours for the jejunum, and 12–30 hours for the ileum, with marked individual variations.

2. An Example of Intubation Studies

Metoprolol is the first drug the absorption of which has been studied all along the GI tract, from the stomach to the caecum [15–18]. Three variants of the intubation technique were used in this investigation.

2.1 Absorption in the Stomach, Duodenum and Jejunum [17]

Five volunteers participated in this experiment. The evening before the study, a triple-lumen tube was positioned fluoroscopically with a perfusion site at the ampulla of Vater, a duodenal aspiration site at the angle of Treitz, and a jejunal aspiration site 30 cm distal to this point. A double-lumen tube was positioned in the stomach with its tip in the antrum (Fig. 1). On the following morning, the gastric content was first continuously aspirated for 1 hour. At the same time, a 20 g/l solution of PEG 4000 in saline was perfused into the duodenum at a flow rate of 2 ml/min. Then, a homogenized meal containing 100 mg of metoprolol and 30 μCi of ^{14}C-PEG 4000 was introduced in the stomach by means of the gastric tube. Thereafter gastric and intestinal contents were sampled every 20 minutes over 4 hours. At the end, the gastric content was aspirated and the stomach rinsed with 200 ml of saline containing 5 g of PEG 4000. At last blood samples were also collected.

The main results of this study were the following:

a) Metoprolol is not absorbed in the stomach: this is demonstrated by the constancy of the metoprolol to ^{14}C-PEG 4000 ratio over 4 hours. In addition, the "apparent" absorption of metoprolol, as calculated by the difference between the amount given and the sum of the amount recovered in the stomach and that lost from the stomach by gastric emptying and sampling over 4 hours, corresponded to 11% of the amount administered. The same calculation gave 7.6% for ^{14}C-PEG 4000.

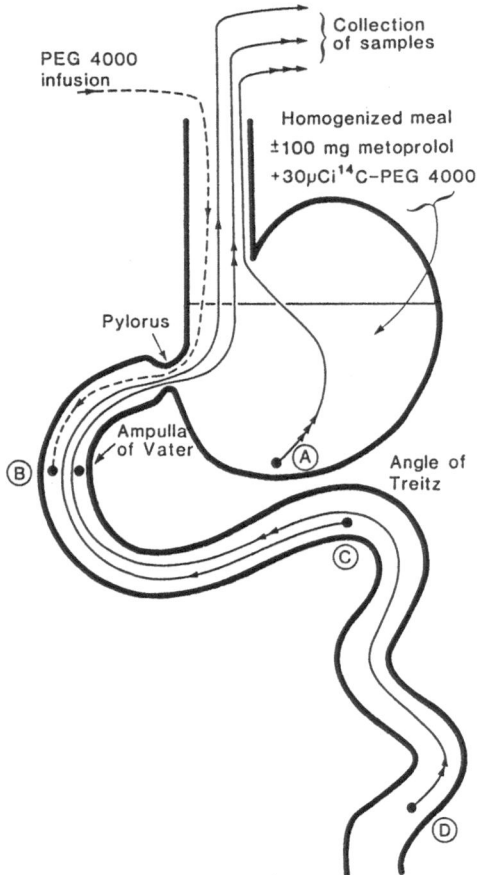

PEG 4000 infusion

Collection of samples

Homogenized meal ±100 mg metoprolol +30μCi^{14}C–PEG 4000

Pylorus

Ampulla of Vater

(B)

(A)

Angle of Treitz

(C)

(D)

Fig. 1
Schematic representation of the position of the tubes within the gastrointestinal tract. Distance from B to C = 20 cm; distance from C to D = 30 cm.
(Reproduced from Brit. J. Clin. Pharmacol., **19**, 97S (1985) with permission of the publisher).

b) There is a linear relationship between the rate of duodenal or jejunal absorption and the rate of delivery to the studied segment. The coefficients of correlation of the two regression lines are 0.909 (n = 62) and 0.932 (n = 44) respectively.
c) The absorption rates are the same in the duodenum and jejunum. The slopes of the regression lines are 0.56 and 0.63 respectively.
d) The metoprolol concentrations in plasma roughly reflect the variations of the absorption rate.

2.2 Absorption in the Jejunum and Ileum [18]

The study consisted of two parts, each of which was carried out over three consecutive days. In the afternoon of the first day, the subjects were intubated with a four-lumen tube incorporating an occlusive balloon. This balloon, once inflated, avoided contamination by endogenous secretions, and reflux of the perfusate above the infusion point. Immediately above the balloon, a tube allowed continuous aspiration of the luminal content. The drug infusion was done immediately below the balloon, and the luminal fluid recovered 30 cm distal to the infusion point (Fig. 2).

On the morning of the second day the perfusion point, checked radiologically, was positioned just beyond the angle of Treitz. At the beginning of the infusion, the balloon was inflated, and its occluding effect checked with bromosulfonphtalein introduced above the balloon with sampling below it.

On the third day, the same procedure was followed with the drug being perfused in the middle part of ileum. The protocol consisted of the following parts: a) an 80 minutes equilibration period during which a saline solution of PEG 4000 was perfused, b) a 60

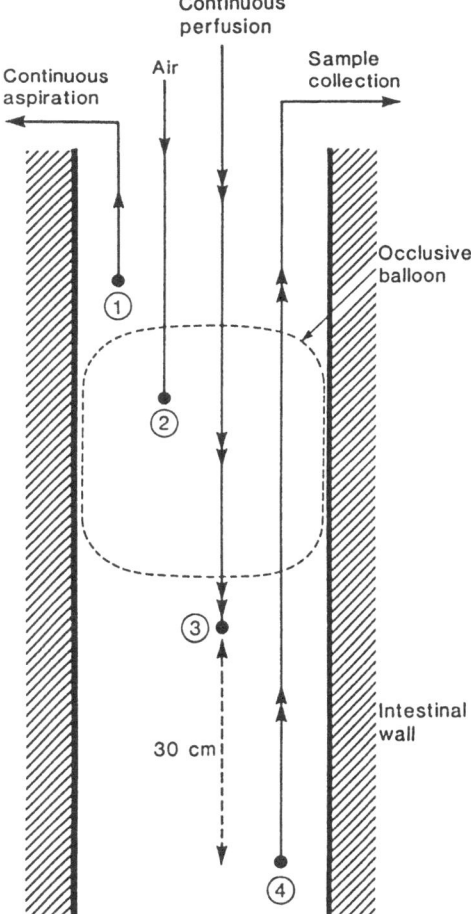

Fig. 2

Schematic reprentation of tubes in the intestine. (Reproduced from Brit. J. Clin. Pharmacol., **19**, 107S (1985) with permission of the publisher).

minutes equilibration period during which a saline solution of metoprolol and marker was perfused, and c) a 80 minutes rinsing period to eliminate metoprolol from the lumen. The last two steps were repeated three times with different concentrations of drug. This part of the study demonstrated:

a) the absorption rate of metoprolol is the same in the jejunum and ileum,
b) there is a linear relationship between the rate of infusion and the rate of absorption,
c) when metoprolol is perfused dissolved in saline, its absorption rate is four times lower than when it is given with a liquid meal.

2.3 Absorption in the Colon [16]

It is not possible to collect representative samples of the luminal content of the colon. For this reason, the absorption rate of metoprolol in the colon was indirectly compared to that in the jejunum. On the first day, in the afternoon, a double-lumen tube was introduced into the intestine. In the morning of the second day, its distal end was positioned under radiological control at a site close to the duodeno-jejunal junction. A metoprolol solution in saline was perfused for 2.5 hours. On the third day, the tube was repositioned with its end located in the caecum and the same perfusion was repeated. Blood samples were collected in the two occasions and the plasma concentration profiles of metoprolol were obtained. They were superimposable and demonstrated that the absorption of the drug is the same in the jejunum and caecum.

2.4 Influence of Food and Digestive Secretions on Metoprolol Jejunal Absorption [15]

To determine whether food or digestive secretions or both increase the absorption rate of metoprolol (see § 2.2.), a special investigation was conducted, which extended over 4 days. On the first day, the subjects were intubated with a four-lumen tube incorporating an occlusive balloon. The perfusion site, below the occluding balloon, was located just beyond the duodeno-jejunal junction. On each of the following three days, one of the following experiment was performed:

1. The balloon was inflated and gastrointestinal secretions were continuously aspirated over the balloon. A saline solution of metoprolol was perfused below the balloon and luminal samples collected 30 cm distally.
2. The balloon was not inflated, allowing gastric, biliary and pancreatic secretions to enter the test segment. The saline solution of metoprolol was perfused at the same site as in 1.
3. The conditions were the same as in 2, but the drug was dissolved in a liquid meal.

In all three experiments, the test segment of jejunum was 30 cm long and the luminal fluid was aspirated continuously. After a 50 min equilibration period, ten successive 10-min samples were collected.

This experiment clearly showed that food, but not digestive secretions, increase the absorption rate of metoprolol in the jejunum. Plasma and urine samples demonstrated that the first-pass metabolism is not modified by the variation of the absorption rate.

3. Conclusion

In the example summarized above, the intubation technique proved to be a useful and efficient technique to explore the gastrointestinal absorption processes of drugs in man. It made it possible — for the first time in the pharmaceutical science — to investigate the absorption of a drug from the stomach to the colon. In addition, it provided a lot of secondary informations about the relationships between the absorption rate and the plasma concentration profile, the role of water movements in drug absorption, the first-pass metabolism as a function of the site of absorption, etc. . . . It permitted the effect of metoprolol on postprandial gastric function to be studied in detail [19].

The same techniques were later on applied to another beta-blocker: oxprenolol, with similar results (to be published), and they are presently adapted to the study of an acidic drug: diclofenac-sodium, which requested the elaboration of some new variants of the intubation technique [20].

Nevertheless, it must be emphasized that the intubation approach is not simple. It requests first a close cooperation between gastro-enterologists with a good know-how of the procedure and pharmacological chemists. It also demands a good selection of the volunteers. It is costly and very time-consuming. Then it must be reserved to the investigation of a few drugs, the absorption of which is worth being investigated in details.

References

[1] J. Hirtz: *Brit. J. Clin. Pharmacol.*, **19**, 77S (1985).
[2] J.C.K. Loo and S. Riegelman: *J. Pharm. Sci.*, **57**, 918 (1968).
[3] J.G. Wagner and E. Nelson: *J. Pharm. Sci.*, **52**, 610 (1963).
[4] A. Gerardin, D. Wantiez and A. Jaouen: *J. Pharmacokin. Biopharm.*, **11**, 401 (1983).
[5] W.D. Abbott and T.G. Miller: *J. Am. Med. Ass.*, **106**, 16 (1936).
[6] S. Hyden: *Ann. Roy. Agr. Coll. Uppsala*, **22**, 411 (1956).
[7] B. Borgström, A. Dahlqvist, G. Lundh and J. Sjovall: *J. Clin. Invest.*, **36**, 1521 (1957).
[8] H.P. Schedl and J.A. Clifton: *J. Clin. Invest.*, **40**, 1079 (1961).
[9] J.S. Fordtran, R. Levitan, V. Bikerman, S.B.A. Burrow and F.J. Ingelfinger: *Trans. Ass. Amer. Physicians*, **74**, 195 (1961).
[10] E.D. Jacobson, D.C. Bondy, S.A. Broitman and J.S. Fordtran: *Gastroenterology*, **44**, 761 (1963).
[11] J.J. Bernier and A. Lebert: *Biol. Gastroenterol*, **4**, 851 (1971).
[12] J.R. Malagelada, G.F. Longstreth, W.H.J. Summerskill and V.L.W. Go: *Gastroenterology*, **70**, 203 (1976).
[13] R. Modigliani, J.C. Rambaud and J.J. Bernier: *Digestion*, **9**, 176 (1973).
[14] S. Hyden: *Ann. Roy. Agr. Coll. Uppsala*, **22**, 139 (1955).
[15] D. Evard, N. Vidon, J. Godbillon, M. Bovet, M. Duval, J.P. Schoeller, J.J. Bernier and J. Hirtz: *Brit. J. Clin. Pharmacol.*, **19**, 119S (1985).
[16] J. Godbillon, D. Evard, N. Vidon, M. Duval, J.P. Schoeller, J.J. Bernier and J. Hirtz: *Brit. J. Clin. Pharmacol.*, **19**, 113S (1985).
[17] G. Jobin, A. Cortot, J. Godbillon, M. Duval, J.P. Schoeller, J. Hirtz and J.J. Bernier: *Brit. J. Clin. Pharmacol.*, **19**, 97S (1985).
[18] N. Vidon, D. Evard, J. Godbillon, M. Rongier, M. Duval, J.P. Schoeller, J.J. Bernier and J. Hirtz: *Brit. J. Clin. Pharmacol*, **19**, 107S (1985).
[19] G. Jobin, A. Cortot, E. Danquechin-Dorval, J. Godbillon, J.P. Schoeller, J.J. Bernier and J. Hirtz: *Brit. J. Clin. Pharmacol.*, **19**, 127S (1985).
[20] P. Dechelotte, P. Ducrotte, J. Godbillon, B. Hecketsweiler, J. Hirtz, P. Hecketsweiler (to be published).

Diskussion

Frage
Sie haben die Absorptionsraten entlang des Gastrointestinaltraktes gemessen. Welche Rolle spielen die Oberflächen der entsprechenden Darmabschnitte und wie werden Unterschiede hinsichtlich der Absorptionsraten wirksam, wenn mit anderen Darmabschnitten verglichen wird?

Antwort
Die Absorption findet vom Ausgang des Schlauches bis zu irgendeinem Ort im Darm statt. Über die dabei beteiligte Oberfläche können keine Aussagen gemacht werden.

Hinweis aus dem Auditorium
Bei ähnlichen Experimenten mit Polyäthylenglykol fand man, daß eine vorhandene Reduktion oder Zunahme der Oberfläche bei der Absorption von Metoprolol keine Rolle spielt.

Frage
Bestehen Unterschiede der Absorption bei konventioneller Untersuchungsmethode und Intubationstechnik, d.h. beeinflussen die Versuchsbedingungen, wie Lage der Sonde, Mahlzeit, Kooperation usw. die Plasmakonzentrationsverläufe?

Antwort
Die Frage ist wegen der bekannten Komplexität der Einflüsse nicht befriedigend zu beantworten. Aus den vorliegenden Einzelergebnissen können keine verallgemeinernden Schlußfolgerungen gezogen werden.

Angemeldete Diskussionsbemerkung Drewe
Beispiel einer Substanz mit einer schlechten Bioverfügbarkeit bei oraler Applikation über eine Sondentechnik, bei der 4 verschiedene Varianten realisiert wurden. Das Präparat wurde im Magen, in der Nähe der Papille oder unterhalb der Treitz'schen Falte appliziert. Eine fünfte Applikation erfolgte mit einer 3 m langen Sonde in den terminalen Ileumbereich. Ein proximales Absorptionsfenster, das aus Vorversuchen postuliert wurde, konnte in diesen Untersuchungen ausgeschlossen werden, da die Plasmakonzentrationszeitverläufe nach der intestinalen Applikation den einer normalen oralen Applikation weitgehend entsprachen.

Frage zur Diskussionsbemerkung Drewe
Welchen Einfluß hatten Löslichkeit, Ionisationsgrad und pH-Wert? Wurden tatsächlich die Absorptionsvorgänge verändert oder nur die Voraussetzungen der Absorption, also z.B. Löslichkeit, Löslichkeitsvolumen modifiziert?

Antwort
Sicher liegen unterschiedliche physiko-chemische Bedingungen bei der Applikation im Magen und im Dünndarm vor. Entlang des Dünndarms sind die physiko-chemischen Bedingungen weitgehend konstant.

Simultaneous Pharmacokinetic and in vivo Gamma Scintigraphic Monitoring in the Development of an Enprofylline-Sustained Release Tablet

J. Ulmius[1], Z.G. Wagner[2], O. Borgå[1], P. Wollmer[3]

[1]AB Draco, [2]Fyzikon AB and [3]Dept of Clinical Physiology, University of Lund; S-22100 Lund

Summary

The in vivo dissolution and absorption of a sustained release enprofylline tablet labelled with Technetium-99m-sulphur colloid was monitored in six healthy subjects in two food regimens by the use of gamma-scintigraphy and drug analysis of plasma and urine samples. The main difference between fed and fasted conditions was in gastric residence time with mean values 3.6 h (fed) and 1.2 h (fasted), whereas the transit time in the small intestine was almost unaffected by food (3.0 verus 3.1 h). In the stomach and the small intestine absorption of enprofylline was governed by the dissolution of enprofylline from the tablet, whereas in the colon the rate-limiting step was absorption. The colon also seemed to be the major absorption site. The results provide a basis for the development of enprofylline sustained release dosage forms.

Introduction

Enprofylline is a new anti-asthmatic xanthine derivative [1]. The short elimination half life (1.5–2 hours) necessitates a sustained release (SR) dosage form for oral maintenance therapy. For the development of such a dosage form, it is essential to have knowledge of the absorption of enprofylline from different parts of the gastrointestinal tract. When given orally as an aqueous solution, enprofylline is absorbed rapidly and completely [2]. After direct administration into the duodenum, a very fast (resembling an i.v. injection) and complete absorption results. When introduced into the colon, enprofylline gives flat and sustained plasma concentration curves and almost complete absorption [2].

The behaviour of a sustained release dosage form of enprofylline throughout the main part of the gastrointestinal tract was studied with the non-invasive technique of gamma-scintigraphy. The position of the dosage form and the in vivo dissolution were determined simultaneously with the plasma levels of enprofylline. Thereby a correlation between position and absorption was established.

13

Materials and Methods

Study Design

The study was carried out on 6 healthy volunteers aged between 25 and 44 years. The study was performed with two regimens, either fasting overnight with breakfast half an hour before tablet administration, or fasting overnight, tablet administration on an empty stomach and continued fasting. For both regimens lunch was served 3 1/2 hours after tablet administration.

Preparation of the Dosage Form

A tablet granulation of enprofylline was sprayed with a Technetium-99m-sulphur colloid solution. Typically 16 g of the granulation was sprayed with 1.2 ml solution with a total activity of 4.2 GBq. The granulation was dried overnight at room temperature. The granulation was then screened and the activity was adjusted to about 30 MBq/g by addition of cold enprofylline granulate. Magnesium stearate was admixed and tablets of nominal weight 440 mg and containing a nominal dose of 300 mg of enprofylline were compressed on a single punch press using 16x7 mm capsule-shaped punches.

The in vitro dissolution test in simulated intestinal or gastric fluid was performed using USP Method II apparatus at 50 rpm and 37 °C. Samples were withdrawn and analyzed for enprofylline using HPLC and for radioactivity using an automatic gamma-counter (LKB-Wallac 1271 Ria-gamma).

Gamma-Scintigraphy

The labelled tablet with an activity of about 10 MBq was administered together with 200 ml of water labelled with about 3 MBq Technetium-99m-sulphur colloid for outlining the stomach. External markers (Co−57) were placed on processus xiphoideus and the lower ribs (subcostal plane) to facilitate repositioning of the subject during imaging. At the moment of ingestion of the tablet and the solution, the subject was standing in front of the gamma-camera (General Electric 400T with a low energy high resolution collimator). The data collection was done on line to a PDP 11/34 computer equipped with a Gamma-11 program. The distribution of activity was stored in a frame consisting of 64 by 64 pixels. Anterior and posterior images, each of 30 s duration, were taken at intervals of 30 minutes. When it was obvious from the images that the tablet had disintegrated the intervals were changed to 60 minutes. From the scintigrams the residence times in the stomach and the transit times through the small intestine were determined. The gastric residence time was taken to be the time when the tablet left the area outlined by the labelled solution. The arrival in the colon was taken to be the time when the movements of the tablet changed from being extended in the small intestine to very small in the colon. Towards the end of the study the radioactivity from the tablet spread in the colon, which also aided the visualization of this organ. The in vivo dissolution from the tablet was determined by monitoring the decrease in radioactivity in a selected area over the tablet. Corrections were applied for background activity, counts arising from release from the dosage form and the solution for outlining the stomach and for radioactive decay. Geometric mean values of the corrected anterior and posterior counts were used in the dissolution plots [3].

14

Pharmacokinetic Studies

Venous heparinized blood samples (5 ml) for plasma preparation were drawn from an antecubital vein before drug administration (blank) and every half hour until 3 hours thereafter, then every hour until 14 hours after tablet administration. One sample was taken at 24 hours. Urine was collected quantitatively in portions for 0−14, 14−24, 24−36 and 36−48 hours after drug administration. Enprofylline in plasma and urine were assayed by an HPLC-method. Bioavailabilty of enprofylline was calculated from both the urine recoveries and the plasma AUC values in relation to an oral solution. The drug plasma concentration profiles were deconvoluted using the method of Langenbucher and Möller [4] to derive the drug absorption data for each subject.

Results and Discussion

A prerequisite for a b.i.d. sustained release preparation of a drug with a half-life of less than 2 hours is that the absorption of the drug occurs during most of the 12 hour dosage interval. During this time a tablet can travel a considerable path-length along the gastrointestinal tract. For the enprofylline SR-tablet the transit time from mouth to ceacum varied between 3 and 8 hours, depending partly on the regimen, partly on individual factors. Consequently, a large fraction of the absorption must take place in the colon to fulfil the above-mentioned criterion.

Fig. 1 shows the radionuclide images of the Technetium-99m-labelled tablet for one typical subject at various times after administration in fed conditions. The outline of the stomach and the colon is depicted. The gastric residence time for this subject was 3 hours and for all six subjects it varied between 3 and 4.5 (mean 3.6) hours during fed conditions. The gastric residence time in fasted conditions was 0.5 hour or less for all but one subject. The small intestinal transit time, taken as the time for arrival at caecum minus the gastric residence time was almost independent of the regimen with mean values of 3.0 and 3.1 hours for the fed and fasted conditions, respectively. Our data agree closely with published values for gastric residence and small intestinal transit times [5].

The SR-formulation of enprofylline is a tablet which functions according to the surface erosion principle. Fig. 2 shows the in vitro dissolution in simulated intestinal fluid of both enprofylline and the label Technetium-99m-sulphur colloid. The dissolution of the two species was parallel with the label being dissolved somewhat faster. This is of course a prerequisite for drawing any conclusions from the in vivo dissolution measurements.

In Fig. 3 all data for the subject shown in Fig. 1 in fed conditions are summarized. In the upper diagram the plasma levels of enprofylline are depicted together with the position of the tablet in the gastrointestinal tract. The lower diagram shows the in vivo dissolution, measured scintigraphically, the cumulative absorbed amount of enprofylline, and also the in vitro dissolution of the technetium label.

As long as the SR-tablet is in the stomach or the small intestine the in vivo dissolution and the absorption curves are superimposed. Since the absorption of a solution of enprofylline is rapid in these parts of the gastrointestinal tract the absorption must be determined by the dissolution of enprofylline from the tablet and/or by gastric emptying.

When the tablet reaches the distal parts of the small intestine the absorption starts to lag behind the dissolution, a state which prevails in the colon as long as the dosage form can be observed. Several mechanisms may explain this behaviour. It is not possible from the

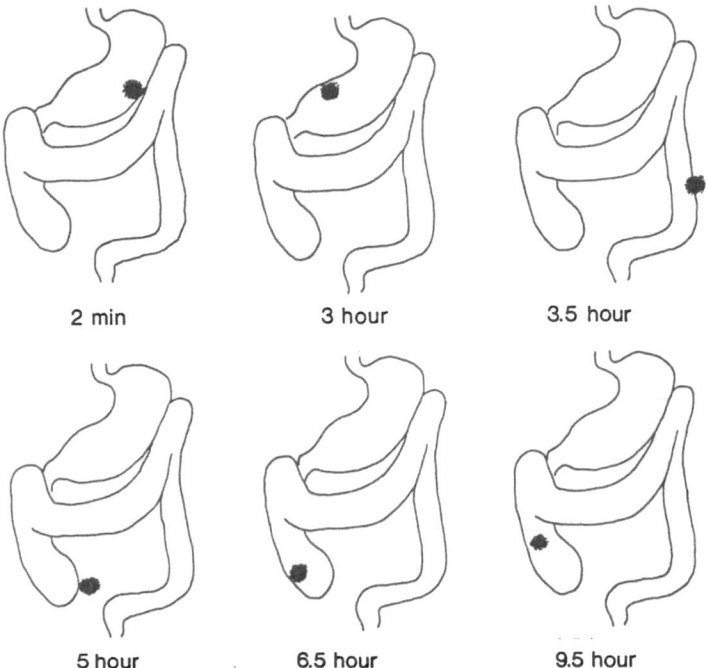

| 2 min | 3 hour | 3.5 hour |
| 5 hour | 6.5 hour | 9.5 hour |

Fig. 1

Radionuclide images of the tablet in the gastrointestinal tract after 2 minutes, 3, 3.5, 5, 6.5 and 9.5. hours after dosing for subject no. 2 during the fed regimen.

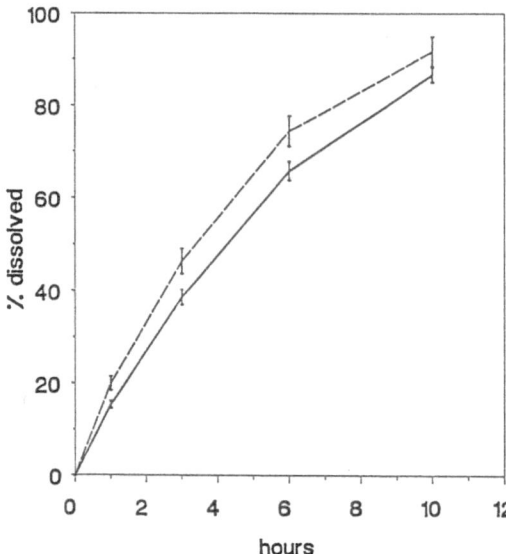

Fig. 2

In vitro dissolution in simulated intestinal fluid without enzymes using USP Method 2 apparatus at 50 rpm and 37°C. Mean ± SEM, n = 12. Solid line: Enprofylline. Broken line: Technetium-99m-sulphur colloid.

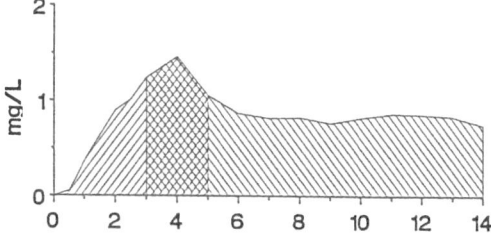

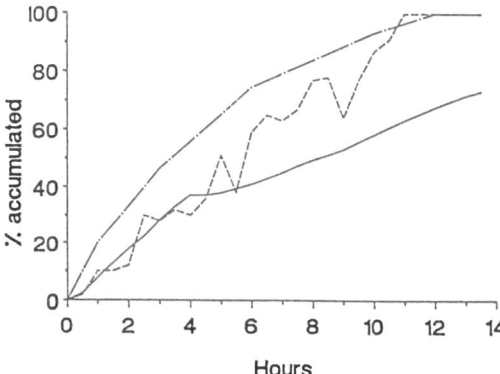

Fig. 3
Data for subject no. 2 in fed conditions. Upper diagram depicts the enprofylline plasma levels and the position of the tablet. Left striped area: time spent in the stomach. Hatched area: time spent in the small intestine. Right striped area: time spent in the colon.

Lower diagram presents per cent of dose dissolved (broken line: in vivo dissolution measured scintigraphically, dash and dotted line: in vitro dissolution of the label) and per cent of dose absorbed (solid line) vs time after tablet administration.

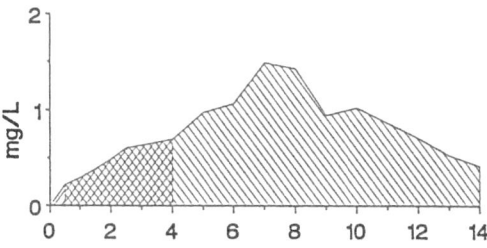

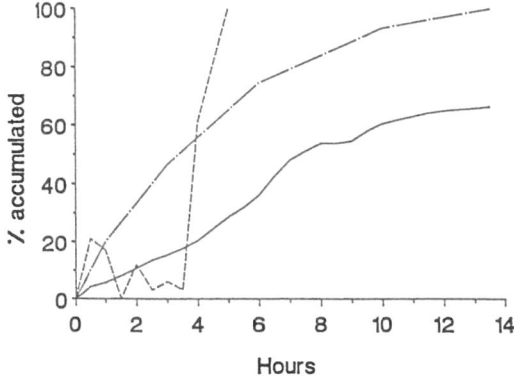

Fig. 4
Data for subject no. 2 in fasted conditions. Same notation as in Fig. 3.

scintigrams to distinguish between dissolution and mere disintegration of the tablet. Hence, the dissolution of enprofylline from the particles from a disintegrated tablet could be the rate-limiting step in the colon. Other possible rate-limiting factors are the transport of dissolved enprofylline to the colon wall and the transport through the colon wall, i.e. the intrinsic absorption rate.

To differentiate between these mechanisms more information is needed. A clue is given in Fig. 4 which shows the data for the same subject in fasted conditions. The tablet leaves the stomach after half an hour and enters the colon after 4 hours. Around this time-point there is a rapid decrease in activity in the tablet and after half an hour the tablet cannot be detected as a unit any longer, which suggests that the tablet has disintegrated. However, there is no corresponding increase in absorption. If the rate-limiting step had been dissolution from small particles or transport to the colon wall, then the observed absorption rate should have been much faster in subjects in whom the tablet had disintegrated, since this process results in a much larger available surface area for dissolution of the substance than for the whole tablet. Therefore, this study indicates that the intrinsic absorption rate of enprofylline in the colon is the rate-limiting step. This is supported by the observed slow absorption rate in the colon for a solution of enprofylline given rectally [2], although it should be noticed that different parts of the colon were involved in the two studies. In no subject could the tablet be detected as a unit in the transverse or the descending colon. The decreasing intestinal water content as the tablet passes along the colon could mean that dissolution or transport of dissolved enprofylline gradually becomes rate-limiting.

The mean curves (Figs. 5 and 6) show the same behaviour as the above presented subject both in fed and fasted conditions, i.e. rate control by the dosage form in the stomach and the proximal small intestine, but in the colon the absorption becomes the rate-limiting step. The absorbed dose when entering the colon is about 50% and 25%, respectively, for the fed and the fasted conditions. The total bioavailability of this enprofylline SR-dosage form is 100% relative to an oral solution (from urine recovery), which means that the colon is the major absorption site. This type of slow but complete absorption in the colon has also been observed for theophylline using a remotely controlled release device for delivering the dose to a predetermined site [6].

Conclusions

The xanthine derivative enprofylline is well absorbed from the small intestine and the colon. The absorption rate in the duodenum is very fast, while it is rather slow in the colon. An SR-dosage form should present rate-limiting dissolution in the stomach and the small intestine, but as long as the dissolution rate is faster than the absorption rate in the colon, there is no need for rate control by the dosage form in this part of the gastrointestinal tract.

The study demonstrates the usefulness of simultaneous pharmacokinetic and in vivo scintigraphic monitoring for investigating the absorption behavior of a drug in a dosage form along the gastrointestinal tract.

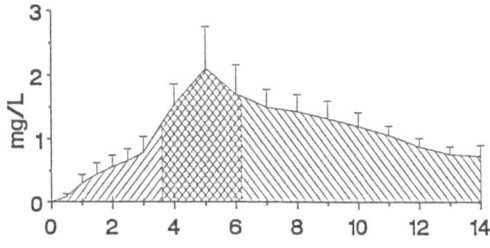

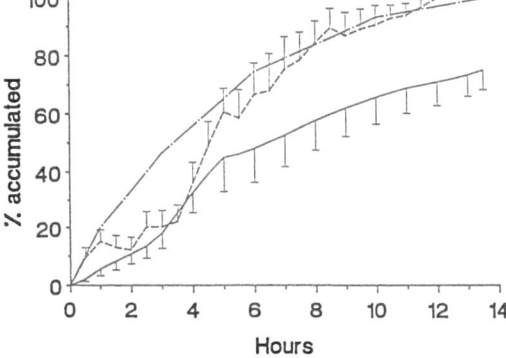

Fig. 5
Mean curves ± SEM, n = 6, for the fed conditions. Same notation as in Fig. 3.

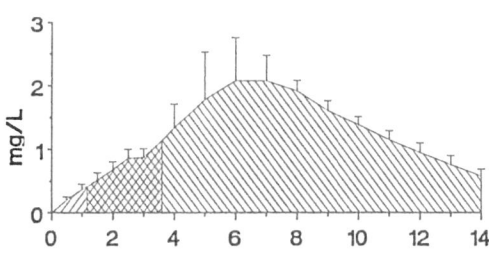

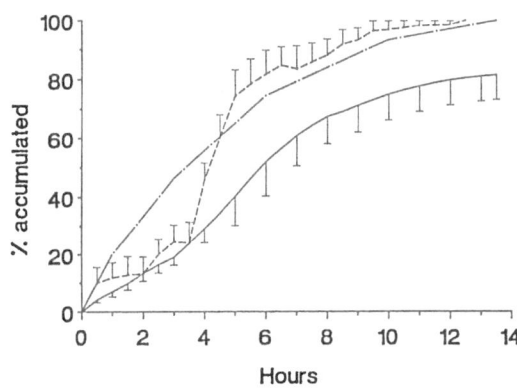

Fig. 6
Mean curves ± SEM, n = 6, for the fasted conditions. Same notation as in Fig. 3.

19

References

[1] C.G.A. Persson and G. Kjellin: Enprofylline, a principally new antiasthmatic xanthine. *Acta Pharmacol. Toxicol.*, **49**, 313–316 (1981).

[2] E. Lunell, K.-E. Andersson, O. Borgå, P.-O. Fagerström, N. Johannesson, G. Kjellin, C.G.A. Persson and K. Sjölund: Absorption of enprofylline from the gastrointestinal tract in healthy subjects. *Eur. J. Clin. Pharmacol.*, **27**, 329–333 (1984).

[3] P. Tothill, G.P. McLoughlin and R.C. Heading: Techniques and errors in scintigraphic measurements of gastric emptying. *J. Nucl. Med.*, **19**, 256–261 (1978).

[4] F. Langenbucher and H. Möller: Correlation of in vitro drug release with in vivo response kinetics I. *Pharm. Ind.*, **45**, 623–628 (1983).

[5] S.S. Davis, J.G. Hardy and J.W. Fara: Transit of pharmaceutical dosage forms through the small intestine. *Gut*, **27**, 886–892 (1986).

[6] A.H. Staib, D. Loew, S. Harder, E.H. Graul and R. Pfab: Measurement of theophylline absorption from different regions of the gastro-intestinal tract using a remote controlled drug delivery device. *Eur. J. Clin. Pharmacol.*, **30**, 691–697 (1986).

Diskussion

Frage
Haben die Dissolutionsrate und ein Substanzabbau im Colon einen Einfluß auf das Ergebnis?

Antwort
Für einen Zerfall des Enprofyllin im Darm liegen keine Hinweise vor.

Frage
Die vorgestellten szintigraphischen Ergebnisse zeigen ein wesentlich unregelmäßigeres Verlaufsprofil als nach Modellberechnungen (Dekonvulutionsmethode) zu erwarten ist. Gibt es hierfür keine Erklärung?

Antwort
Es muß ein Einfluß der Darreichungsform angenommen werden.

In vivo Dissolution and Absorption Kinetics of Sustained-Release Theophylline, Studied with Stable Isotope Methodology

J. Caldwell, S.A. Hotchkiss

Department of Pharmacology, St. Mary's Hospital Medical School,
London W2 1PG, U.K.

Summary

It is essential to assess the absorption characteristics and bioavailability of drugs from sustained-release formulations. In the case of theophylline, there are two schools of thought as to the correct method for the conduct of such studies. The rate constant of drug elimination must be determined, which may be done either by a cross-over design with a reference conventional preparation or from the terminal phase of the log plasma concentration-time curve. The former method may be criticized in the light of the known intra-subject volatility of theophylline half-life, while there are considerable analytical difficulties in the use of the latter approach. We have adopted an experimental design which overcomes these problems by coadministering a sustained-release formulation (Uniphyllin) together with stable isotope (^{15}N) labelled theophylline in solution as the reference material to 7 healthy volunteers. Gas chromatography-mass spectrometric analysis permitted the separate determination of both forms (^{14}N and ^{15}N) of theophylline. Log plasma concentration-time curves were plotted for each form, and the absorption characteristics of the ^{14}N-theophylline contained in the sustained-release formulation determined by the Wagner-Nelson method and numerical deconvolution (the point-area technique). The K_{el} of ^{14}N-theophylline was decreased compared with ^{15}N-theophylline (longer half-life) so that the absorption kinetics were more correctly determined using the ^{15}N-pharmacokinetic parameters. Both mathematical methods of analysis gave comparable results for the absorption profiles for the sustained-release formulation.

This method has allowed the first direct evaluation of the absorption and bioavailability of theophylline from a sustained-release preparation. Problems caused by inter- or intra-subject lability in theophylline K_{el} are eliminated, resulting in the valid use of much smaller numbers of subjects. Only one dosing session is required, with only one set of blood samples. Comparison of *in vivo* absorption profiles with the results of *in vitro* dissolution tests reveals that while the mean data are comparable, there does occur considerable inter-subject variation in absorption kinetics, which may hinder direct extrapolation of in vitro dissolution data to the patient situation.

Introduction

Theophylline (1,3-dimethylxanthine) has a pharmacological profile which makes it suitable for the treatment of asthma and a variety of other obstructive airways disorders. Its therapeutic usefulness is hampered by its poor pharmacokinetic properties, which include a narrow therapeutic window of plasma concentrations, and a short and highly variable plasma elimination half-life [1, 2, 3]. Little therapeutic benefit is seen from plasma concentrations of less than 8−10 µg/ml, whilst sustained levels in excess of 20 µg/ml are associated with an increased risk of toxicity. The extensive clinical use of theophylline at the present time is a consequence of the widespread availability of plasma level monitoring services and the existence of numerous sustained-release preparations of the drug. These formulations are used in order to maintain plasma concentrations within the therapeutic range, avoid toxicity and give acceptable dosing intervals for patient use.

As with all drug delivery systems, the kinetics of absorption and bioavailability of theophylline must be established from sustained-release formulations. A number of methods are available for such studies, the majority of which require a knowledge of the elimination rate constant of the drug in question [4, 5]. In the case of theophylline there are considerable difficulties in measuring this reliably, and opinion is divided as to how this should be done. One school of thought opines that the elimination rate of theophylline can be determined directly from the terminal decline phase of plasma theophylline concentrations [6]. However problems may be encountered here over the definition of the true terminal phase from sustained-release preparations. Firstly, these preparations may give rise to "trickle absorption", and secondly the low plasma levels of drug at the time of "terminal" elimination phase may challenge the accuracy of analytical methodologies. As an alternative it has been suggested that the elimination rate constant may be determined with reference to a conventional preparation in a cross-over design [7]. Volunteers receive, on separate occasions in random order, conventional and sustained-release preparations of the drug. This approach is rendered problematical in the case of theophylline by the extreme lability of elimination rate which may be encountered within individual subjects: intra-subject variation of up to 60% has been reported [2].

The study to be described in this paper is intended to determine the true absorption kinetics and bioavailability of theophylline from a sustained-release formulation, by co-administration of the sustained-release preparation with a reference solution of ^{15}N-theophylline. The separate assay of ^{14}N and ^{15}N-theophylline in plasma thus allows a calculation of the true elimination rate constant (from the ^{15}N-theophylline data) and hence the true absorption kinetic parameters of the ^{14}N-theophylline from the sustained-release formulation.

Methods

Seven healthy non-smoking male volunteers, ages 21−38 years, body weight 65−95 kg, gave their informed consent for participation in this study, which was approved by the Ethics Committee of St. Mary's Hospital and Medical School. The subjects abstained from all methylxanthine containing foods and beverages for 3 days prior to and during the study. Following an overnight fast, each subject was given 100 mg ^{15}N-theophylline dissolved in 200 ml water, the solution being used to swallow a 400 mg sustained-release theophylline tablet (Uniphyllin, Napp Laboratories). Venous blood samples were collected either from an indwelling cannula or venepuncture from the antecubital fossa, at regular intervals up to 30 h after drug administration. Plasma levels of theophylline were determined by HPLC, using an automated version of the method of Cotgreave and Caldwell [8]. The separate assay of ^{14}N and ^{15}N-theophylline was achieved by capillary gas chromatography-mass spectrometry with selected ion monitoring: for this assay theophylline was converted to its pentafluorobenzyl derivative [9]. The correlation coefficient for the determination of theophylline by these two methods was greater than 0.98. The absorption kinetics of theophylline were calculated either by the Wagner-Nelson method [4] or by the numerical deconvolution method of Vaughan & Dennis [5]. The dissolution of theophylline from the sustained-release tablet was determined by the British Pharmacopoieal method [10].

Results and Discussion

Fig. 1 shows plots of the mean theophylline plasma concentrations versus time for both ^{14}N and ^{15}N-theophylline after the administration of both substances to the volunteers. This clearly shows the rapid absorption of the ^{15}N-theophylline from solution as compared with the slower absorption of ^{14}N-theophylline from the sustained-release tablet. The elimination rate constant for the reference solution is slightly greater than that observed for ^{14}N-theophylline from the sustained-release tablet. The areas under the plasma level time curves are approximately proportional to the doses administered. Table 1 summarizes various of the pharmacokinetic parameters describing the disposition of the two forms of theophylline in the panel of 7 subjects. Where appropriate, values have been corrected for the difference in doses between the two preparations. As expected there are significant differences between the two preparations in both C_{max} and T_{max}. The elimination rate constant for ^{15}N-theophylline is slightly but significantly greater than that for the ^{14}N form, and there are comparable changes in the elimination half-life. The areas under the plasma concentration time curves are also significantly different when corrected for dose, with smaller values being seen for the ^{14}N-theophylline derived from the sustained-release formulation.

The kinetics of absorption of theophylline from the sustained-release formulation were determined by both the Wagner-Nelson and point area methods, using the elimination kinetics of ^{15}N-theophylline for reference. There were no significant differences between the results obtained by the two methods of calculation. The % absorbed vs. time plot (Fig. 2) for the sustained-release formulation reveals firstly the occurrence of considerable inter-individual variability between the subjects, and secondly that absorption is biphasic, with a second, slower phase commencing some 6h after administration. The recent studies of Staib et al. [11], involving the use of a remotely controlled device for the release of drugs in different regions of the gastrointestinal tract, have shown that the rate, but not extent, of absorption of theophylline is variable along the gut. Thus, the rate of absorption becomes slower as the drug is presented to lower and lower parts of the gut, and it may be that the slower absorption phase seen from 6h after administration of Uniphyllin is a consequence of the transit of theophylline into the intestine. The biphasic absorption pattern thus seems to be a characteristic of theophylline per se rather than the particular dose form examined here.

The in vitro dissolution characteristics of theophylline from Uniphyllin tablets has been investigated by the British Pharmacopoieal method, into 0.6% HCI for the first hour

23

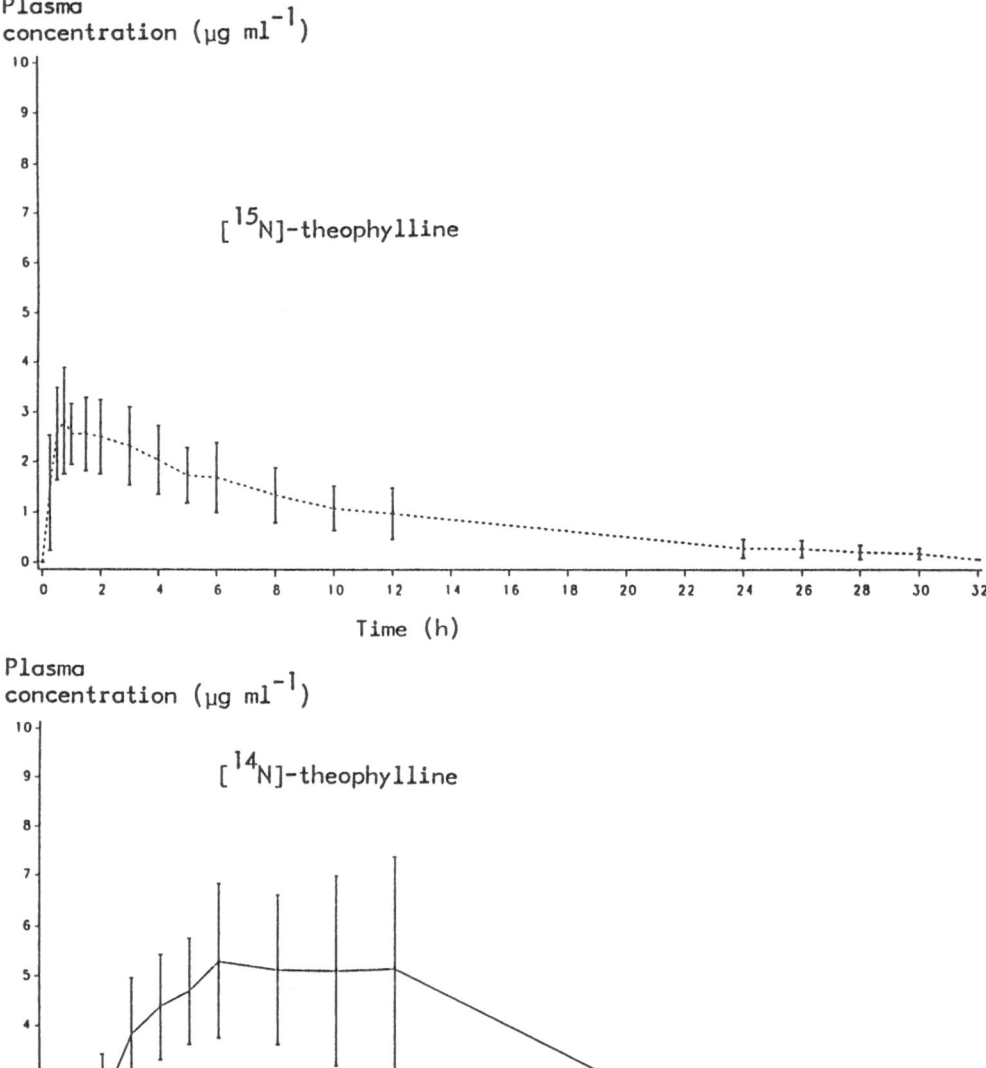

Fig. 1
Mean plasma concentration-time profiles of (^{14}N)- and (^{15}N)-theophylline in seven subjects.

Table 1. Pharmacokinetic parameters describing the plasma concentrations of (^{14}N) theophylline given in solution (^{15}N) and in sustained-release tablets (^{14}N).

	^{14}N	^{15}N
$C_{max}^{(ug\,ml^{-1})}$	6.2 ± 2.1 (15.5 ± 5.3)*	3.1 ± 1.0 (31.0 ± 10.0)*
T_{max}(h)	9.1 ± 2.5*	0.8 ± 0.5*
K (h^{-1})	0.101 ± 0.019*	0.113 ± 0.021*
t½ (h)	7.1 ± 1.4*	6.3 ± 1.2*
AUC (ug h ml^{-1})	111.5 ± 40.9 (278.8 ± 102.3)*	31.0 ± 12.7 (310.0 ± 127.0)*

* Significantly different (p < 0.05) betweem preparations.
Figures in brackets are per g dose of theopylline

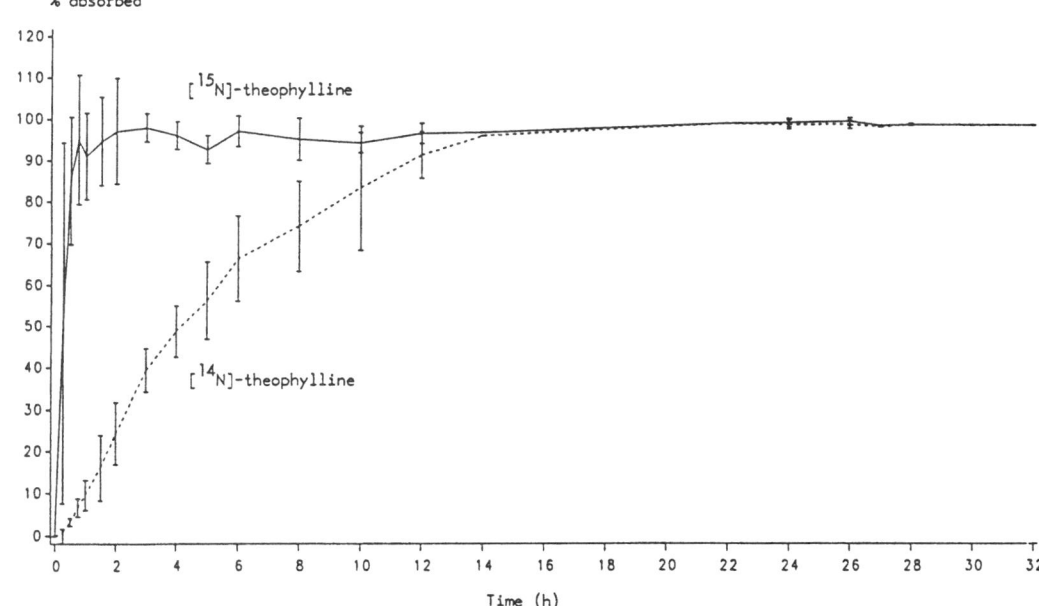

Fig. 2
Mean percent theophylline absorbed-time plots for conventional (^{15}N) and sustained-release (^{14}N)theophylline.

followed by 1.5% Na HCO$_3$ up to 8 h. This has shown a zero-order release pattern of theophylline, with some 11% being released per hour.

It is of interest to consider the correlation between the release of theophylline from Uniphyllin in vivo and in vitro, especially in view of the various uses to which in vitro dissolution data are put. Fig. 3 shows clearly the deviation of this relationship from an exact correlation, and its variation with time during the experiment. The substantial interindividual variation in the extent of absorption with time is also apparent.

In conclusion, therefore, this study has for the first time allowed a direct investigation of the absorption characteristics and bioavailability of theophylline from a sustained-release formulation. The experimental approach adopted has overcome the various problems resulting from traditional cross-over designs. Although it is generally recognized that the experimental design adopted here will reduce the numbers of subjects as compared with cross-over designs, it is important to note that there occurs substantial inter-subject variation in absorption kinetics not attributable to experimental design, and the number of subjects must be sufficient for the proper assessment of such variability. This type of experimental design makes fewer demands on the subjects, but the need for stable isotope-labelled compounds and mass spectrometric analysis adds very significantly to the cost of the study. Last, but by no means least, the availability of the present

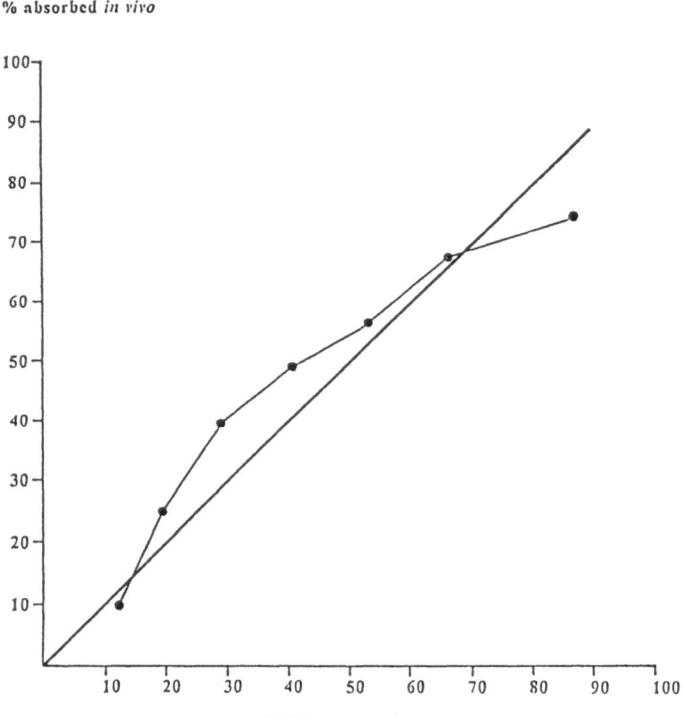

Fig. 3

Relationship between % absorbed in vivo and % released in vitro of theophylline from Uniphyllin tablets over 8 hours.

techniques has shown that in vitro dissolution data, obtained by a typical pharmacopoieal method, may not be readily extrapolated to human subjects.

Acknowledgements

This work was supported by grants from Napp Laboratories Ltd. We thank Dr. E. Bailey and Dr. P.B. Farmer for assistance with mass spectrometry, and Prof. R.L. Smith for continued encouragement of work in this area.

References

[1] P.A. Mitenko, R.I. Ogilvie: Rational intravenous doses of theophylline. *N. Engl. J. Med.* **289**, 600–603 (1973).
[2] R.A. Upton, J.F. Thiercelin, T.W. Guentert, S.M. Wallace, J.R. Powel, L. Sansom, S. Riegelman: Intra-individual variability in theophylline pharmacokinetics: Statistical verification in 39 of 60 healthy young adults. *J. Pharmacokinet. Biopharm.* **10**, 123–134 (1982).
[3] M. Weinberger, L. Hendeles, L. Wong: Relationship of formulation and dosing interval to fluctuation of serum theophylline concentration in children with chronic asthma. *J. Pediatr.* **99** (1), 145–152 (1981).
[4] J. Wagner, E. Nelson: Percent absorbed time plots derived from blood levels and/or urinary excretion data. *J. Pharm. Sci.* **52**, 610–611 (1963).
[5] D.P. Vaughan, M. Dennis: Mathematical basis of point-area deconcolation method for determining in vivo input functions. *J. Pharm. Sci.* **67** (5), 663–665 (1978).
[6] J.G. Wagner: Effect of using an incorrect elimination rate constant in application of the Wagner-Nelson method to theophylline data in cases of zero order absorption. *Biopharm. Drug Disp.* **5**, 75–83 (1984).
[7] M. Weinberger, L. Hendeles, L. Bighley: The relationship of product formulation to absorption of oral theophylline. *N. Engl. J. Med.* **299**, 852–857 (1978).
[8] I.A. Cotgreave, J. Caldwell: Comparative plasma pharmacokinetics of theophylline and ethylenediamine after the administration of aminophylline to man. *J. Pharm. Pharmacol.* **35**, 378–382 (1983).
[9] E. Bailey, P.B. Farmer, J.A. Peal, S.A. Hotchkiss, J. Caldwell: Analytical methodology to determine stable isotopically labelled and unlabelled theophylline in human plasma using capillary gap chromatography-mass spectrometry. *J. Chromatog.* In press.
[10] I.A. Cotgreave,J. Caldwell: Comparative pharmacokinetics of theophylline and ethylenediamine following single and repeated doses of a sustained-release aminophylline preparation to volunteers. *J. Pharm. Pharmac.* **37**, 618–621 (1985).
[11] A.H. Staib, D. Loew, S. Harder, E.H. Graul, R. Pfab: Measurement of theophylline absorption from different regions of the gastro-intestinal tract using a remote controlled drug delivery device. *Eur. J. Clin. Pharmacol.* **30**, 691–697 (1986).

Diskussion

In einem Kommentar zu den Ergebnissen wird festgestellt, daß die intraindividuelle Variabilität wesentlich kleiner ist als die interindividuelle.

Frage
Kann hieraus geschlossen werden, daß mit konventioneller Technik ausreichend gute Ergebnisse erzielt werden?

Antwort
Entsprechend den FDA-Richtlinien sind wegen der sehr unterschiedlichen Einflüsse auf die Theophyllin-Kinetik differenzierende Untersuchungen wie die vorgestellten notwendig.

Course of Development of the HF-Capsule — Variations and Method-Related Typical Findings

O. Schuster, B. Hugemann

PAZ GmbH, Bereich Arzneimittelentwicklung, D-6230 Frankfurt/M. 80

Summary

Knowledge on the absorption of compounds along the GI-tract is important information for the development of sustained release formulations, in diagnosis and with respect to open questions in the nutrition.

In order to examine the absorption characteristics in animal and man we developed a HF-capsule releasing compounds at any predetermined region of the GI-tract.

The localisation of the HF-capsule within the GI-tract is X-ray controlled and the spontaneous release is initiated by a short impuls of a HF-generator.

With respect to the absorption characteristics the examined drugs may be divided into the following groups:

- No difference of absorption quotes along the whole GI-tract. These substances are suitable for SR-formulations with an extended release characteristic.
- Decrease of bioavailability from proximal to distal parts of the gut. These substances may be suited for a limited retard-effect.
- Increase of bioavailability from proximal to distal parts of the intestine. These substances should be incorporated in formulations with a spontaneous release in the colon or in the ileocecal region.

These evaluations show that substance-related specific absorption windows in the GI-tract cannot be ignored.

1. Introduction

In the development of galenic formulations, in diagnostics and the nutritional sciences it is important to have information about the absorption characteristics of the substances from different parts of the GI-tract.

Especially when controlled-release formulations are developed the question often arises whether the aimed prolongation of the drug's efficacy can be assured under therapeutic conditions and with a minimum of side-effects. This is a pre-requiste for, among others, the optimization of the pharmacokinetics of slow release preparations. From the pharmacokinetic point of view the active principle should be liberated and absorbed during its gastrointestinal passage to the same extent as it is eliminated from the biophase or is metabolically inactivated. The release-characteristics can only be adapted to the therapeutic needs, when:

28

- the transit-characteristics of the test-formulation under therapeutic conditions are known,
- the extent and rate of absorption of the substance from the sites of the GI-tract where the substance is released are known.

These transit-investigations are performed with X-ray or scintigraphic methods.
For the experimental evaluation of the extent and rate of absorption from the different sites of the GI-tract, several techniques for an enteral application are available, e.g. intubation techniques, chemical coatings regulated by the pH or dissolution time, endoscopic techniques and positioned release capsules [1].

2. Positioned Release Capsules

From the mentioned techniques for the application of drugs to different sites of the GI-tract, in this presentation only the application of positioned release capsules will be discussed in more detail.

2.1 Development Phases

Capsules which released the active principle after a pre-selected period of time have already been used some decades before. Because of the variations in the transit-times these are not suitable to release substances in a chosen area. Magnetic release-mechanisms never got beyond a pilot testing phase.
A suitable remote controlled capsule was described when studies were performed to investigate the absorption of iron from the gut [2]. In this capsule a piston which restricts the reservoir with the drug, is kept tensioned by two springs. The release procedure starts after heating up all metallic parts by high frequency and a melting pearl of Wood's metal melts at 47°C. By this the two springs are disengaged and the piston pushes out the drug − solution. To heat up the metal parts, a high transmitting power of the high frequency source is necessary which leads to a local warming. A capsule for diagnostic purposes (after Grenier), recently presented in the rainbow press, is capable of picking up signals with sensors in the intenstine and sending these to an external receiver. In addition substances may also be released [3]. The release mechanism depends on the dissolution rate of a gelatine layer despite the built-in sophisticated electronic equipment.
Thus this capsule offers no advantages over simple gelatine capsules with respect to substance applications. Nevertheless with this technique physiologic changes after the release of the substance in the intestine can be observed, if appropriate sensors are available. Positioned release capsules like the "Endoradiosonde" (Heidelberger Kapsel), which is used exclusively for diagnostic purposes, will not be presented here.

2.2 Technique and Function of the High-Frequency Capsule (HF-Capsule)

For the convenient, stress-free application of substances at any location of the GI-tract a remote controlled capsule was developed [4]. This capsule has no built-in electrical energy source. The energy needed for starting the drug release is supplied from an external high-frequency transmitter. Due to the exact resonance tuning of the receiver integrated in the capsule, the trigger pulse for the opening mechanism can be kept at a very low energy level. The principle of the HF-capsule is illustrated in Fig. 1; the capsule consists of a smooth plastic case with a length of 28 mm and a diameter of 12 mm, which remains unchanged during the transportation through the GI-tract. In one half of the capsule the drug-device is localized. This part consists of a small latex balloon, which can be filled with the aid of normal hypodermic needles or injection syringes via an adapter. The maximum filling volume is 1 ml; solutions, suspensions and solids are suitable as fillings. In the other half of the capsule the release mechanism is located. The capsule is actuated when a high frequency field is applied from outside the body and an oscillating circuit (coil and capacitor) within the capsule absorbs energy. This absorbed energy heats up a heating wire which melts a nylon thread holding a spring with a small needle under tension. Disengaging the spring, the water-resistant central part of the capsule is pierced, the balloon gets punctured and thus releases immediately the drug. The release mechanism is triggered by a commercial 27 MHz high frequency generator and a special designed ring antenna. Figure 2 depicts the HF-capsule filled with micro-pellets (left) and a solution (right).

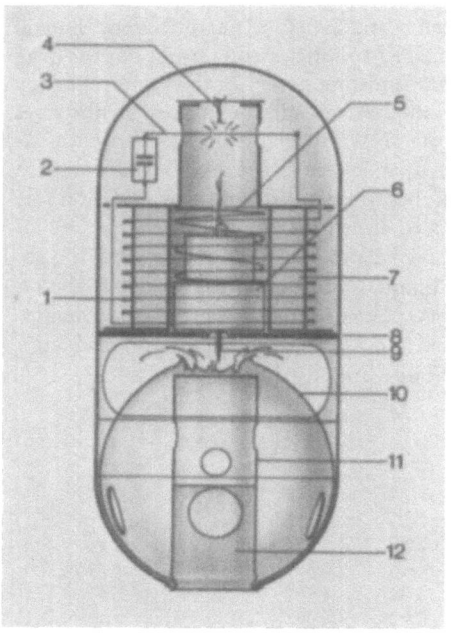

Fig. 1
Scheme of the HF-capsule

1 oscillating circuit	7 cylinder liner
2 capacitor	8 separation wall
3 heating wire	9 small steel needle
4 nylon thread	10 latex container
5 spring	11 holder for 10)
6 plunger	12 plug

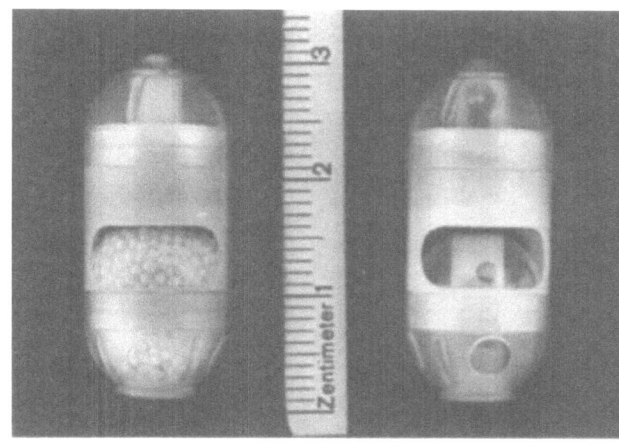

Fig. 2
HF-capsule filled with micro-pellets (left) and a solution (right).

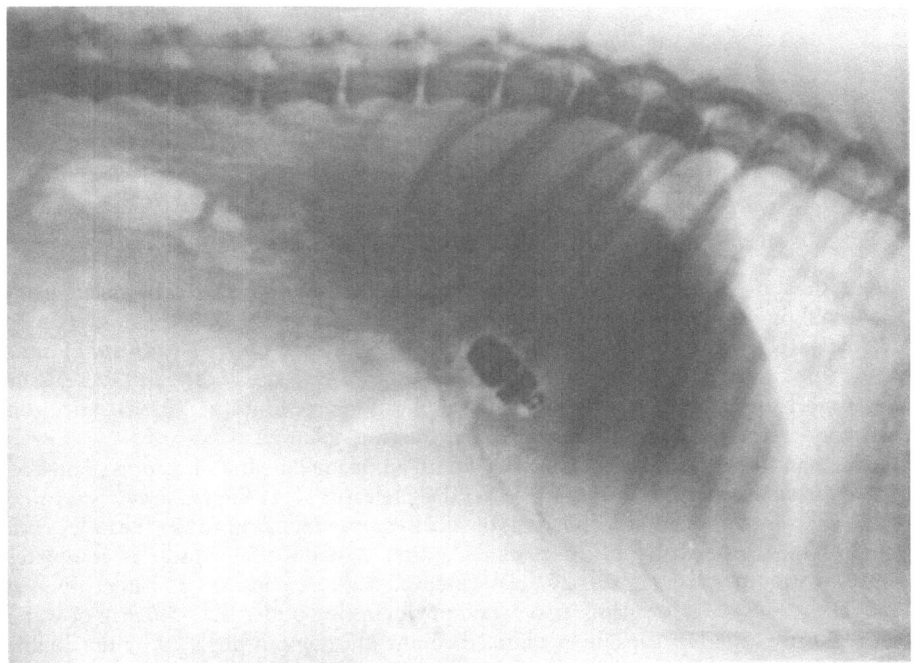

Fig. 3
X-ray picture of an HF-capsule filled with an opaque medium taken before drug-release in a beagle.

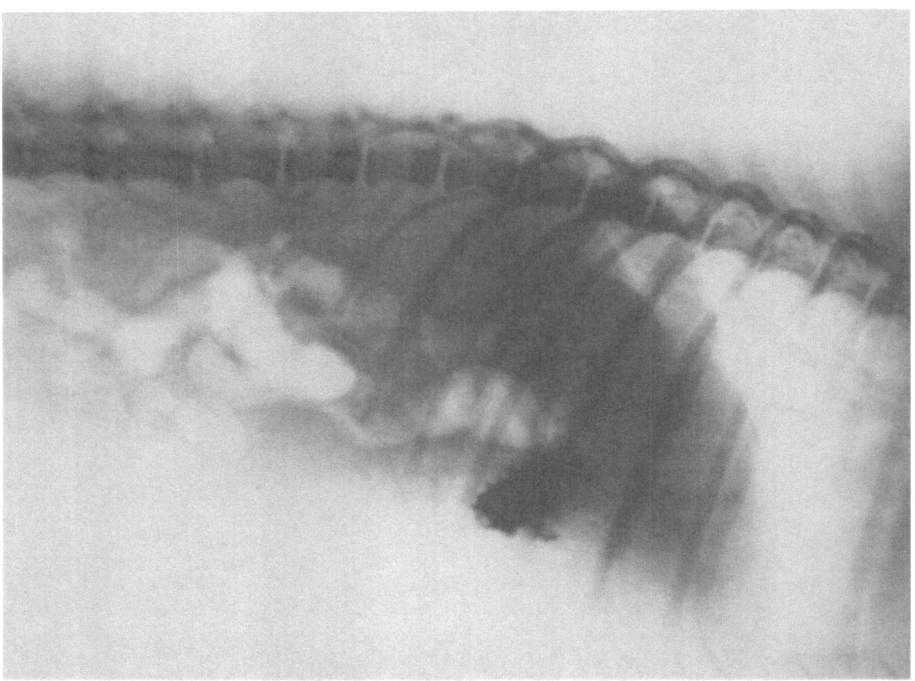

Fig. 4
X-ray picture of an HF-capsule filled with an opaque medium taken 10 seconds after drug release in a beagle.

2.3 Localization of the HF-Capsule and Release of the Substance

The localization of the capsule and demonstration that the capsule has been actuated is performed by a short-time x-ray screening and a transducer. As the capsule consists of metallic parts it can be easily recognized. Before it was used for a first time in humans, the capsule was optimized in pilot studies with dogs. The shape of the capsule, seals and release mechanism were varied until an easy application procedure, safe gastro-intrestinal transit and a fast liberation of the active principle was achieved.

Figures 3 and 4 show an HF-capsule filled with an opaque medium in a dog's non-contrasted intestine before and 10 seconds after drug release. These figures show that, forced by the pressure of the bursting balloon, the drug escapes rapidly through the holes in the frame of the capsule. Already 1–2 minutes after actuation the capsule is completely empty. A spontaneous release may also achieved with suspensions and micro-pellets. Frequently, releasing-problems arise when powders clog under the influence of water. Figure 5 shows the HF-capsule in a human colon. The colon is depicted by the double-contrast-technique. By special radiologic techniques it is possible to localize the capsule without application of an opaque substance; therefore pharmacokinetic interactions between drug and the opaque medium can be excluded.

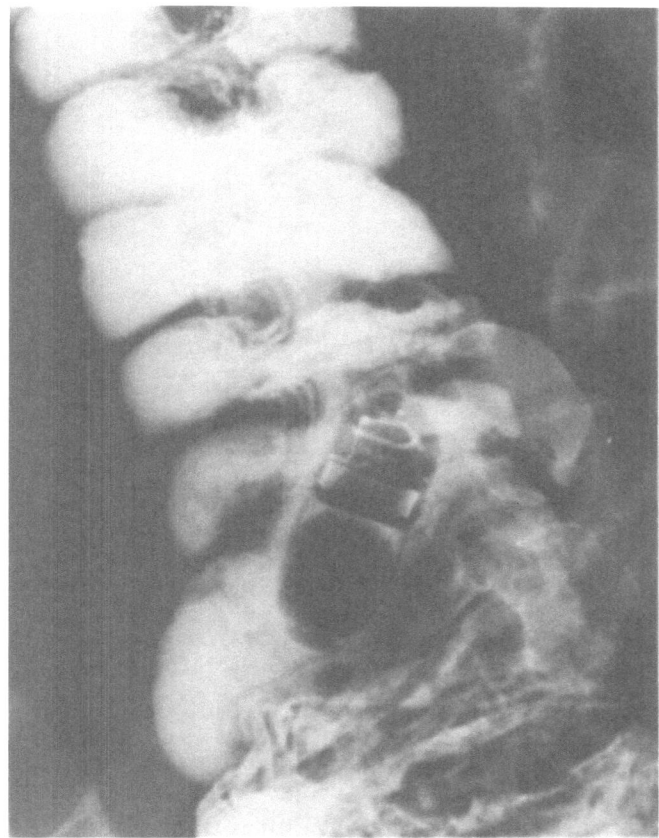

Fig. 5
HF-capsule filled with an opaque medium located in the human colon
(double-contrast-technique)

3. Results from Pre-Clinical and Clinical Pharmacokinetic Studies

From the material collected up to now some examples are presented which should demonstrate the compound-dependent variations of absorption from various sites of the GI-tract:

— in beagle-dogs two ^{3}H- and ^{14}C-labelled test preparations with similar molecular structures were released at the same time in the upper duodenum and the distal ileum. An evaluation of the blood-levels shows that the ^{3}H-labelled compound exhibits a pronounced decrease of the AUC between duodenum and ileum (Fig. 6). The ^{14}C-labelled compound however shows a less pronounced difference in the AUC but a shift of the peak blood-levels of about 2 hours (upper duodenum) to 4 hours (distal ileum).

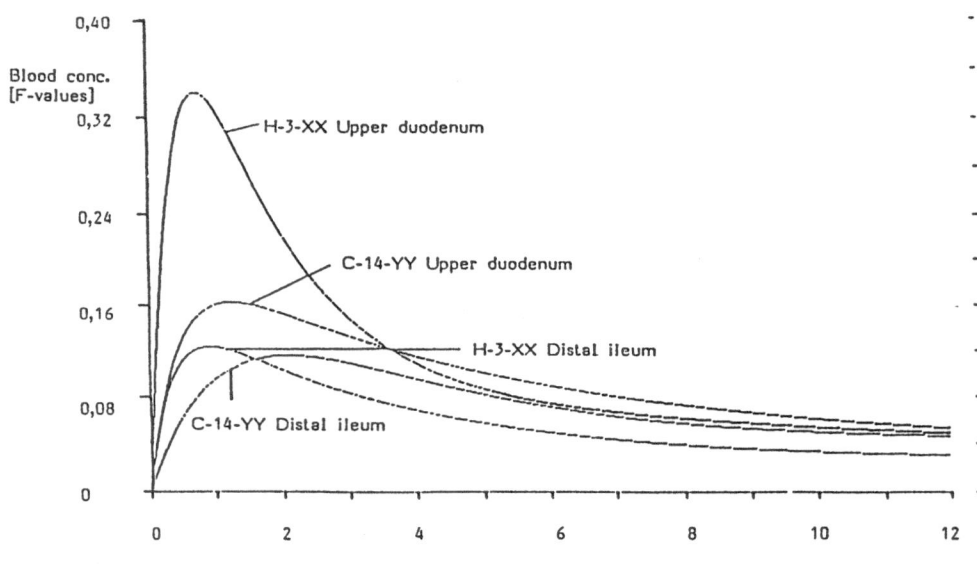

Fig. 6

Blood concentration-time-plot of two labelled (^{3}H − xx and ^{14}C − yy) compounds after drug release in the upper duodenum or distal ileum.

- the first study with humans, performed with the compound AR-L 115, developed by Thomae, revealed that after releasing the substance in the stomach and duodenum the same extents of absorption were achieved. This extent of absorption was much lower when the release was performed in the colon [5].
- pronounced differences were observed after the release of 300 mg of allopurinol in the duodenum as well as the middle and lower jejunum [6] (Fig. 7). In contrast to the serum levels of allopurinol, those of its active metabolite oxipurinol showed much smaller differences. These results demonstrate the importance of the pharmacokinetic parameters of metabolites in studies investigating absorption. Therefore, the kinetics of active metabolites like oxipurinol, should be evaluated, too. − Similar pronounced differences of the absorption characteristics in the GI-tract were found for furosemide [7].
- contrary to the substances mentioned above, metoprolol showed no differences in extent and rate of absorption from the stomach and colon [8]. After the release of 100 mg in the stomach and colon of 10 volunteers, no significant differences concerning c_{max}, t_{max}, $t_{1/2}$ and AUC were detected (Tab. 1). These results substantiate the findings obtained from studies with intubation techniques [9]. Similar absorption characteristics in studies with the HF-capsule were observed with indomethacin, theophylline [10] and isosorbide-5-nitrate [11].
- a compound with a very low absolute bioavailability (2%) after p.o. administration showed an increase of bioavailability by a factor of 10−20(!) (Fig. 8). After p.o. administration of 200 mg the same AUC's were found as after the release of 15 mg in the colon.

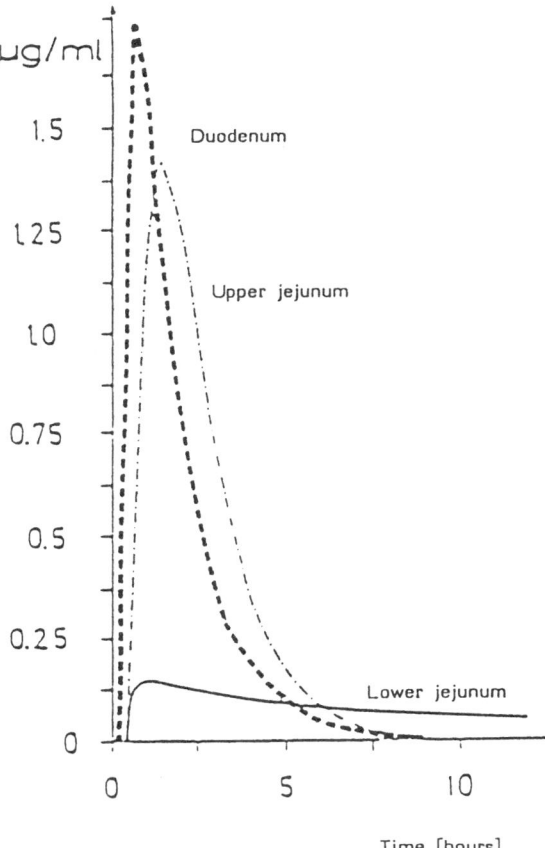

Fig. 7
Serum allopurinol concentrations in ten volunteers after release of 300 mg in the doudenum, middle jejunum and lower jejunum.

Table 1: Absorption of metoprolol in 10 volunteers after release of 100 mg in the stomach and colon, respectively

Dosage	c_{max} (nmol/l)	t_{max} (h)	$t_{1/2B}$ (h)	$AUC_{(0-8h)}$ (nmol/l × h)	$F_{rel.}$
Tablet	574.6 ± 93.6	1.94 ±0.23	3.71 ±0.39	2648 ± 535	1.0
HF-capsule	581.5 ± 81.4	1.38 ±0.27	4.21 ±0.72	2715 ± 542	1.09 ±0.7

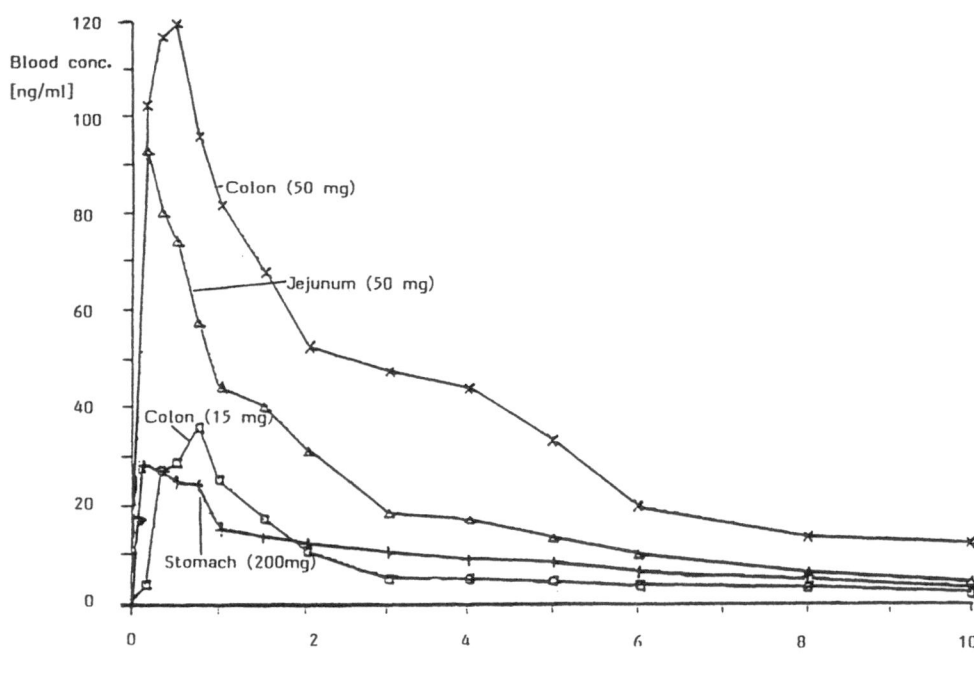

Fig. 8

Release of a compound with a high pre-hepatic first-pass-effect in the colon (50 and 15 mg), jejunum (50 mg) and stomach (200 mg).

Conclusion

The extent and rate of drug absorption from all sites of the GI-tract can be investigated with the HF-capsule.

The compounds investigated up to now may be divided into several different groups with respect to their absorption characteristics:

— drugs with a high extent of absorption exclusively from the stomach or the upper parts of the duodenum are of only limited use for the development of retard preparations. At best they may be suited for a very limited retard-effect, because one has to take into account a reduced bioavailability. One should also look for the main metabolites when comparative bioavailability studies are performed, as changes in the metabolic clearance will lead to erroneous statements concerning the extent of absorption.

— substances which show no differences in extent and rate of absorption passing from stomach to colon are, a priori, suitable for the development of controlled release formulations with markedly prolonged dissolution characteristics.

— substances with a high systemic availability in the colon should be released in the colon.

These evaluations show that drug related specific absorption windows in the GI-tract can not be ignored. It is not possible make a statement whether these different absorption characteristics at different sites of the GI-tract depend on the dissolution of the compound in the intestine's lumen or the penetration/crossing of the mucosal membrane. If metabolites are not determined too, false conclusions may be obtained because of changes of the intestinal metabolic conditions.

References

[1] J. Hirtz: The gastrointestinal absorption of drugs in man: a review of current concepts and methods of investigation. *Br. J. clin. Pharmac.* **19**, 77S–83S (1985).

[2] A. Hemmati: Die Bestimmung des Resorptionsortes von Eisen im Intestinalkanal mit einer ferngesteuerten Darmkapsel. *Dtsch. med. Wschr.* **93**, 1468–1472 (1968).

[3] H.-J. Raabe: Die Pille, die auch Fotos macht. *Bunte* **10**, 50–51 (1986).

[4] B. Hugemann, O. Schuster: *Deutsche Patentschrift* DE 2928477 C3 (1982).

[5] A. Zimmer, W. Roth, B. Hugemann, W. Spieth, F.W. Koss: A novel method to study drug absorption. Evaluation of the sites of absorption with a capsule for wireless controlled drug liberation in the GI tract. *Proc. First Europ. Congr. Biopharm. Pharmacokin.*, Clermont-Ferrand, Vol. 2, Technique et Documentation, pp. 211–214, Paris.

[6] O. Schuster, M. Haertel, B. Hugemann, J. Gikalov, O. Schiemann, H. Fenner: Untersuchungen zur klinischen Pharmakokinetik von Allopurinol. *Arzneim. Forsch./Drug Res.* **35**, 760–765 (1985).

[7] E.H. Graul, D. Loew, O. Schuster: Voraussetzung für die Entwicklung einer sinnvollen Retard- und Diuretika-Kombination. *Therapiewoche* **35/38**, 4277–4291 (1985).

[8] U.E. Jonsson, A. Sandberg: Absorption study of metoprolol with a positioned release capsule. *Second Int. Conf. on Drug Absorption, Rate Control in Drug Therapy*, Edinburgh (1983), Abstr., p. 68

[9] J. Godbillon, D. Evard, N. Vidon, M. Duval, J.P. Schoeller, J.J. Bernier, J. Hirtz: Investigation of drug absorption from the gastrointestinal tract of man. Metoprolol in the colon. *Br. J. clin. Pharmac.* **19**, 113 S – 118 S (1985)

[10] D. Loew, A.H. Staib, N. Rietbrock, E.H. Graul, J. Kollath, S. Harder, B. Hugemann, O. Schuster: Direct measurement of drug absorption along the intestinum of man. Studies with furosemide and theophylline. *III World Conf. on Clin. Pharmacol & Therapeutics*, Stockholm, July 27 – Aug. 1, 1986; *Acta Pharm. Tox.*, Suppl. 1986, p. 82, Abstr. 195

[11] A. Wildfeuer, H. Laufen, R. Dölling, G. Pfaff, B. Hugemann, H.E. Knoell, O. Schuster: Bedeutung galenischer Formen für die orale Therapie mit antianginösen Substanzen. *Therapiewoche* **36**, 2996–3002 (1986)

Diskussion

Hinweis aus dem Auditorium
Es wird darauf hingewiesen, daß Pharmakokinetik und Metabolismus bei dieser Methode bereits bekannt sein sollten, um Irrtümer bei der Interpretation zu vermeiden. Bei der Beurteilung der Resorption muß berücksichtigt werden, daß die Substanz bei tieferen intestinalen Applikationsorten an der Leber vorbeigeschleust wird und demzufolge die metabolisierte Fraktion verändert sein kann. Dies erklärt auch den Befund einer scheinbar schlechteren Absorption der zitierten Substanz durch einen außerordentlich hohen first-pass-Metabolismus. Bei der Colonapplikation ist dann die Resorption im Verhältnis zu höheren Darmabschnitten scheinbar verbessert. Ferner ist nicht nur der hepatische first-pass-Effekt, sondern auch der intestinale first-pass-Effekt bei solchen Untersuchungen zu berücksichtigen.

Frage
Welchen Einfluß hat die Verweilzeit der Kapsel in bestimmten Darmabschnitten? Sind mögliche Schwierigkeiten bei der eindeutig definierbaren Lokalisation der Kapsel im Magen-Darm-Trakt wegen der zeitlichen Bedingungen möglicherweise kompensierbar?

Antwort
Die Kapsel wurde mehrfach in Gewicht und Form verändert. Sie wurde insbesondere schwerer gemacht, so daß die Passage durch den Magen gleichmäßiger erfolgt. Durch gleichzeitige Verabreichung von Antiemetika kann ferner eine Art Synchronisierungseffekt auf die Passagegeschwindigkeit der Kapsel erreicht werden, was jedoch bei pharmakokinetischen Untersuchungen wegen möglicher Substanzinteraktionen meistens unerwünscht ist.

Die substanzspezifische chronopharmakologische Variabilität kann durch zeitversetzte Applikation der HF-Kapseln reduziert werden, so daß die Substanzfreisetzung in den zu untersuchenden Bereichen des Magen-Darm-Traktes etwa zu gleichen Tageszeiten erfolgen kann.

Frage
Liegen systematische Untersuchungen über die Ergebnisvariablität vor und können an die Kapsel Druckfühler angebracht werden?

Antwort
Bisher nicht. Die Streuungen, die bei den Ergebnissen auftreten, sind wesentlich geringer als bei der Anwendung des therapeutischen Oros-Systems, wie aus Untersuchungen am Hund hervorgeht. Bei diesen Untersuchungen bleiben nämlich die Oros-Systeme häufig in der Magenfalte liegen, woraus außerordentlich variable Passagezeiten resultieren. Der Betrieb von Druckfühlern wäre nur beim zusätzlichen Einbau eines Senders möglich.

Frage
Wie sicher ist die Entleerung der Kapsel und welcher Zeitraum wird benötigt?

Antwort
Das hängt von der Art der Füllung ab. Bei Feststoffen können Schwierigkeiten auftreten, bei Pellets ist die Freigabe schon wesentlich besser und bei Flüssigkeiten gibt es überhaupt keine Probleme. Die Entleerung erfolgt innerhalb von Sekunden bis wenigen Minuten.

Evaluation of the Colonic Drug Absorption in Patients with an Artificial Intestinal Stoma and by Colonoscopy in Normal Volunteers

K.-H. Antonin, P. Bieck

Human Pharmacology Institute, Ciba-Geigy GmbH
D-7400 Tübingen

Summary

Absorption of single doses of oxprenolol (80 mg) and of diclofenac-Na (100 mg) administered by colonoscopy into the cecum and the left flexure of the colon was compared with that after oral dosing in healthy volunteers. Plasma concentration/ time profiles of both drugs after oral and colonic dosing followed similar time courses. Oxprenolol reached maximal levels within 2 hours. Mean peak concentrations were lower after colonic compared with oral dosing. From the areas under the concentration-time curves (AUC) the relative bioavailability (BAV_{rel}) was calculated. The mean BAV_{rel} of oxprenolol was 80% after colonic application versus oral administration. Oral and colonic administration of diclofenac-Na resulted in comparable peak plasma concentrations and AUCs. The apparent BAV_{rel} of diclofenac-Na ranged from 50−110% with a mean of 80%.

The absorption of oxprenolol delivered from an oxprenolol OROS® 16/260 was studied in six patients with artificial stomata of the transversal colon. In the morning one oxprenolol OROS® was introduced together with 20 ml water into the distal part of the stoma. Oxprenolol saliva and urinary concentrations were measurable in all patients.

The recovery of oral clioquinol in urine and intestinal contents was studied in patients with a stoma of the terminal ileum or of the colon. The fecal recovery of the drug was highest in patients with ileostomy (90%) and lowest in those with colostomy (50%). The urinary recovery was correspondingly lowest in patients with ileostomy (10%) and highest in those with colostomy.

Drug absorption by the colonic mucosa can be investigated in patients with an intestinal stoma if no stenosis is present or in healthy volunteers after intracolonic administration during colonoscopy. Measuring saliva concentrations of lipophilic drugs with a constant ratio of saliva:plasma concentration may be sufficent for the first evaluation of pharmacokinetics in severely ill patients thus preventing unnecessary blood loss.

Introduction

In the past the absorptive function of the human colon has been studied mainly in connection with the transport of water, electrolytes and ammonia across the mucosa [1]. Relative little attention has been given to drug absorption in this segment of the human gut. This is because most drugs after oral administration in a rapid-release dosage form are completely absorbed from the upper intestinal tract and will not reach the large bowel. In humans mean transit time from mouth to cecum is 3−7 h [2, 3] while that through the entire gut exceeds 20 h [4−6].

In recent years pharmaceutical research has been directed towards the development of special sustained-release dosage forms. These new formulations deliver drugs at constant rate along the entire gut, thus avoiding peak blood concentrations and related adverse effects. A special type of sustained-release formulation is the osmotic drug delivery system (OROS®). The drug is contained within a semi-permeable membrane (Fig. 1). Water from the gut is drawn through the membrane by osmosis, dissolves the drug and forces out the resulting solution through a tiny laser-drilled exit hole. OROS® dosage forms are characterized in terms of their release-rate and total drug content: a 16/260 OROS® system contains 260 mg of drug which is released at a rate of 16 mg/h [7,8]. If the drug release exceeds 7 h parts of the dose will have to be absorbed in the colon. Bioavailability might be restricted by the inability of the colon to absorb the drug. Therefore, it is of great importance to learn whether and to what extent drugs can be absorbed by the colonic mucosa.

Several techniques − such as indirect methods, colonic intubation and more recently high frequency capsules − are available to study colonic drug absorption in man [9]. We have performed colonoscopies in healthy volunteers and took advantage of artificial stomata of the distal gastrointestinal tract in patients to study drug absorption from different colonic segments. In two colonoscopic studies we investigated the colonic absorption of the beta-adrenergic blocker oxprenolol and the nonsteroidal anti-inflammatory drug diclofenac-Na in healthy volunteers. In two studies with patients with intestinal stomata we examined the colonic absorption of oxprenolol and clioquinol. The results have been reported and discussed earlier [10−13]. In this overview the results are presented briefly and the methods discussed.

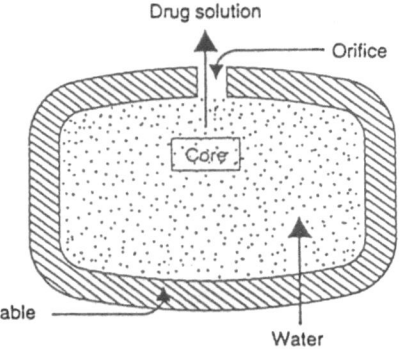

Fig. 1
Cross-section of a typical osmotic drug delivery system (OROS®).

Materials and Methods

The study protocols were approved by an Ethics Committee and informed written consent was obtained from each subject.

Colonoscopic Studies

a) Volunteers

Two studies were performed with six male volunteers each. In the first study (oxprenolol) the age ranged between 23−31 years (mean 29 years) and the body weight between 67−97 kg (mean 77 kg). In the second study (diclofenac-Na) the age was between 20−30 years (mean 26 years) and the body weight between 67−94 kg (mean 87 kg).

All subjects were healthy according to clinical examination and haematological and biochemical screening. None had a history of asthma, allergy or gastrointestinal disease. There were no known contraindications to the administration of beta-receptor blocking or anti-inflammatory drugs. No other medications were allowed for one week before and during the trial.

b) Procedures

At 8 a.m. on the day before colonoscopy each subject swallowed a laxative (X-Prep®, Mundipharma Limburg, West Germany; containing 30 ml standardized extract of senna pods with 150 mg of senna glycosides A und B). On the same day only liquid meals were allowed until 2 p.m.. From this time until 10 p.m. the volunteers had to drink water or tea in large quantities (2−3 l). Thereafter all volunteers fasted until the colonoscopy. One hour before endoscopy an enema (containing 1000 ml of water with 20 g magnesium sulfate) was applied. No premedication or sedative was administered. The procedure was performed with a CF-LB 3 R colonoscope (Olympus) in the Endoscopy Unit of the Department of Internal Medicine, University Tübingen.

The drugs were mechanically pulverized and suspended in 5 ml water and exposed to ultrasound for 10 min. The suspension was applied as a bolus through a thin catheter via the instrumentation channel of the endoscope and was followed by 20 ml water. The drugs were administered into the region of the cecum (n = 3), and of the left flexure (n = 3) (Fig. 2).

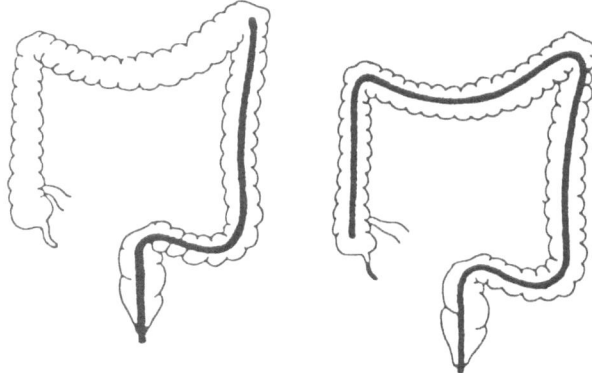

Fig. 2
Illustration of drug application into the region of the left flexure (n = 3; left) and into the cecal region (n = 3; right).

c) Study design

The absorption was first measured after oral administration. After an overnight fast the volunteers took 80 mg oxprenolol (1 tabl. Trasicor® 80) or 100 mg diclofenac-Na (2 tabl. Voltaren® 50) with 100 ml water at 8.00 a.m. Two hours later a standard breakfast was given. Blood samples were collected for 24 or 8 h, resp. Blood was placed into Na-EDTA containing tubes, centrifuged immediately and plasma stored at −20°C until analysis.

After a drug-free interval of at least one week absorption was measured after administration by colonoscopy of 80 mg oxprenolol (1 tabl. Trasicor® 80) or 100 mg diclofenac-Na (2 tabl. Voltaren® 50). Blood samples were collected as described. In subj. 6 administration of oxprenolol into the left flexure of the colon was repeated 13 weeks later.

Studies with Stoma Patients

In two studies the absorptive capacity of the colon was investigated in patients with intestinal stomata. There were no pathological findings in the remaining gastrointestinal tract as shown by clinical examination, endoscopy or x-ray. Their hepatic and renal function were within normal limits.

In the third study nine patients (Table 3) with end ileostomy (n = 2) or end colostomy (n = 7) were given 250 mg clioquinol (1 tabl. Entero-Vioform®) orally with 100 ml of water in the morning after an overnight fast. Urine samples were collected in 12 h inter-

Table 1. Comparison of pharmacokinetic data of oral versus colonic application of 80 mg oxprenolol

Volunteer no.	Site of colonic adminis- tration	Oral application			Colonic application			
		C_{max} [ng/ml]	t_{max} [h]	AUC_{0-24} [ng·h·ml^{-1}]	C_{max} [ng/ml]	t_{max} [h]	AUC_{0-24} [ng·h·ml^{-1}]	BAV_{rel} [%]
1	c	662	1.02	1294	202	0.25	627	48
2	c	429	0.50	791	304	2.00	880	111
3	c	193	1.00	355	76	2.02	288	81
4	lf	435	0.50	707	193	0.50	339	48
5	lf	918	0.50	2447	630	0.70	1396	57
6	lf	304	1.00	1070	1527[1]	0.50	6895[1]	644
	lf				403[2]	0.50	1572[2]	147
mean ± SD		490±262		1111±729	301±195		850±538	82±40
median			0.75			0.50		

c = cecum
lf = left flexure
[1] first administration (values are not used for the calculation of the means)
[2] second administration

Table 2. Comparison of pharmacokinetic data of oral versus colonic application of 100 mg diclofenac-Na

Volunteer no.	Site of colonic adminis- tration	Oral application			Colonic application			BAV_{rel} [%]
		C_{max} [μg/ml]	t_{max} [h]	AUC_{0-8} [μg·h·ml^{-1}]	C_{max} [μg/ml]	t_{max} [h]	AUC_{0-8} [μg·h·ml^{-1}]	
1	c	1.09	3	1.88	1.46	0.50	1.66	88
2	c	1.08	2	2.35	1.73	0.50	2.24	95
3	c	5.51	1	5.22	0.99	0.50	2.87	54
4	lf	1.03	3	1.77	1.59	0.25	1.94	109
5	lf	0.84	3	1.96	1.26	0.50	1.84	94
6	lf	4.45	2	5.36	2.62	0.25	3.09	57
mean±SD		2.34±2.08		3.09±1.72	1.61±0.56		2.27±0.59	83±22
median			2.5			0.50		

c = cecum
lf = left flexure

Table 3. Cumulative urinary and intestinal excretion of clioquinol (C) after acute oral administration of 250 mg to patients with ileostomy or colostomy

Patient no.	Age [y]	Sex	Diagnosis	Surgical therapy	Intestinal excretion (free C) [% dose]	Urinary excretion (free + con- jugated C) [% dose]
1	21	m	Ulcerative colitis	Ileostomy	86	5
2	48	m	Abdominal trauma	Ileostomy	93	17
mean	35				90	11
3	84	f	Rectosigmoidal carcinoma	Colostomy (transverse colon)	45	42
4	78	m	Diverticulitis	Colostomy (transverse colon)	–	15
5	74	f	Diverticulitis	Colostomy (transverse colon)	67	30
6	68	f	Rectal carcinoma	Colostomy (sigmoid colon)	49	38
7	74	f	Rectal carcinoma	Colostomy (sigmoid colon)	57	14
8	63	f	Rectal carcinoma	Colostomy (sigmoid colon)	47	42
9	51	m	Anorectal fistula	Colostomy (sigmoid colon)	–	29
mean	70				53	30

Table 4. Oxprenolol concentrations in saliva and urinary excretion after colonic application of one 16/260 oxprenolol OROS®

Patient no.	Age [y]	Sex	Diagnosis	Saliva concentrations C_{max} [ng/ml]	t_{max} [h]	AUC_{0-24} [ng·h·ml^{-1}]	Urinary excretion (free + conjugated) [mg/36 h]
1	51	m	Diverticulitis of the sigma	317	5.0	3056	—[1]
2	58	m	Colitis ulcerosa, Ca of the sigma	63	12.0	871	9.8
3	72	m	Perforation of the sigma	437	8.0	4533	0.6
4	46	f	Diverticulitis of the sigma	69	5.0	635	11.8
5	56	m	Ca of the rectum	70	5.0	839	8.0
6	59	m	Ca of the rectum	128	12.0	2149	12.5[2]
mean±	57			181	7.4	2014	7.6
SD				159		1552	4.9

[1] urine not collected
[2] not included in calculation because urine was collected from 12–36 h.

vals and intestinal contents in 6 h intervals up to 4 days after dosing. Volume and weight were measured and aliquots stored at −20 °C until assayed.

In the fourth study 6 patients (Table 4) with a loop stoma of the transversal colon were investigated. In the morning one oxprenolol OROS® 16/260 was introduced with 15 ml 0.9% NaCl solution into the distal part of the stoma. Oxprenolol concentrations in saliva and urine were measured to prevent unnecessary blood loss in the patients. Saliva and urine were collected for 24 h and 36 h, resp.

Drug Assays

Oxprenolol concentrations in plasma, saliva, and urine were measured using a modified gas chromatographic method [14].

Diclofenac-Na plasma concentrations were determined by a HPLC method [15].

Clioquinol concentrations in intestinal contents and urine were analyzed by gas chromatography [16].

Data Analysis

Peak plasma or saliva concentrations (C_{max}) and times to peak (t_{max}) were assessed from the individual plasma or saliva concentration-time curves. Areas under the plasma or saliva concentration-time curves (AUC) were estimated by the trapezoidal rule. Relative bioavailability (BAV_{rel}) was assessed by comparing areas under the curve after colonic application with oral application.

Results

Colonoscopy was generally well-tolerated by the subjects. The time required to reach the cecum was 5–20 minutes (mean 11 min). Fluoroscopy was used only rarely for straightening the sigmoid under difficult conditions. X-ray control could be avoided in most investigations.

a) Colonoscopic study with oxprenolol

The individual results (C_{max}, t_{max} and AUC_{0-24}) after oral and colonic administration are given in Table 1 and the mean plasma profiles for both applications are illustrated in Fig. 3.

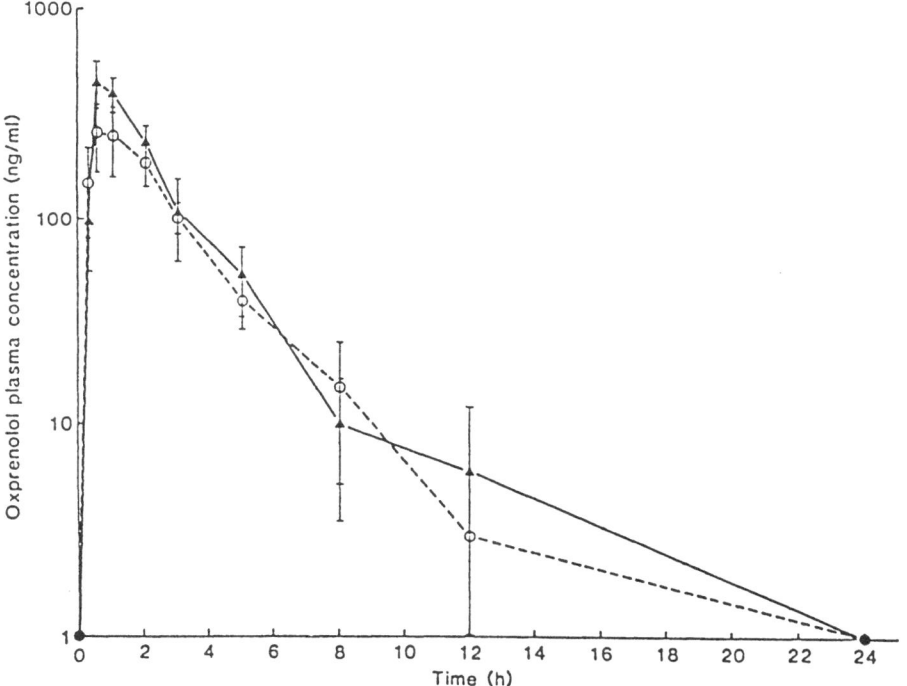

Fig. 3

Plasma concentration time curves after oral (▲——▲) and colonic (○– – – –○) application of 80 mg oxprenolol. Mean ± SEM (n = 6).

Oxprenolol concentrations were measurable in all subjects after oral and colonic administration. There is a considerable interindividual variation in absorption as judged by C_{max} (oral: range 193–918 ng/ml; colonic: range 76–1527 ng/ml) and by t_{max}. The peak concentrations after drug administration were achieved between 0.5 h to 1 h (oral) and between 0.25 to 2 h (colonic), respectively. The AUC_{0-24} varied between 355 and 2447 ng·h·ml^{-1} (oral) and between 288 and 6895 ng·h·ml^{-1} (colonic).

In 5/6 volunteers C_{max} and in 4/6 volunteers AUC were smaller after colonic administration. In subj. 6 C_{max} and AUC were repeatedly greater after colonic application than after oral dosing. The relative bioavailability of oxprenolol (BAV_{rel}) from the large bowel compared with the oral bioavailability ranged from 48% to 644%. When the first data from volunteer 6 were excluded, the mean BAV_{rel} was calculated to be 82% [10].

b) Colonoscopic study with diclofenac-Na

The individual results (C_{max}, t_{max} and AUC_{0-8}) after oral and colonic administration are given in Table 2 and the mean plasma concentration-time curves are given in Fig. 4.

Diclofenac concentrations were measurable in all subjects after oral and colonic application. The amount absorbed after application to the cecum is not different to that after application to the left flexure. Again considerable interindividual variation was found. Oral and colonic administration resulted in comparable mean peak plasma concentrations (C_{max} oral: range 0.84–5.51 μg/ml; colonic: range 0.99–2.62 μg/ml) and similar areas under the plasma concentration time curves between 0 and 8 hours, (AUC_{0-8} oral: range 1.77–5.36 μg·h·ml^{-1}; colonic: range 1.66–3.09 μg·h·ml^{-1}). The relative bioavailability (BAV_{rel}) of diclofenac from the colon compared to the oral form ranged from 54% to 109% (mean of 83%; Table 2) [13].

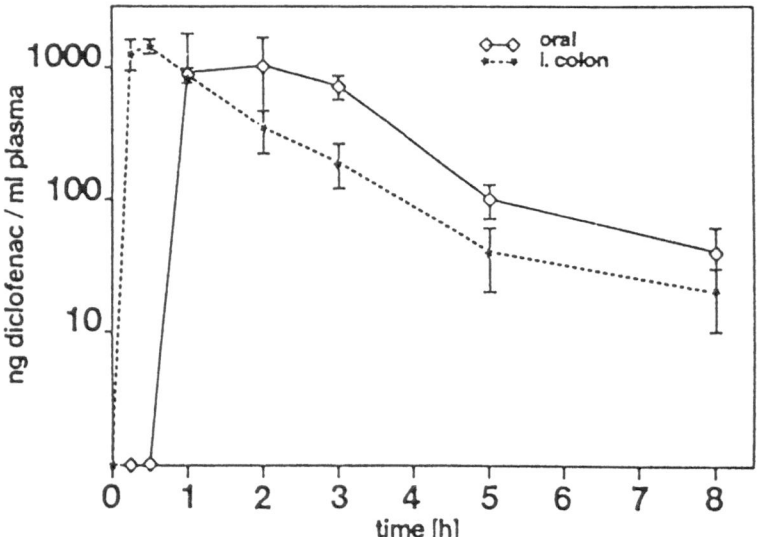

Fig. 4
Plasma concentration time curves after oral and colonic application of 100 mg diclofenac-Na. Mean ± SEM (n = 6).

c) Study in patients with end stomata with clioquinol

The urinary and intestinal excretion of clioquinol is summarized in Table 3 and presented in Fig. 5. In patients with end ileostomy 90% of the given clioquinol dose was recovered in the stool, collected from the stoma. In urine 11% of the dose was recovered. In patients with end colostomy 53% of the clioquinol dose was recovered from the stoma. The mean urinary elimination was 30% of the amount given. There was no essential difference in clioquinol excretion between patients with transverse colostomy and sigmoid colostomy [12].

d) Study in patients with loop stomata with oxprenolol OROS®

The individual results (C_{max}, t_{max} and AUC_{0-24}) are given in Table 4. Individual and mean saliva concentrations are illustrated in Fig. 6 and urinary concentrations in Fig. 7.
After colonic application of one oxprenolol OROS® the drug was detected in saliva and urine of all patients. There was a 7fold difference of saliva concentrations between lowest and highest C_{max} and AUC values. C_{max} values ranged between 63 and 437 ng/ml and AUC values between 635 and 4533 ng·h·ml^{-1}. Mean oxprenolol concentrations in saliva declined 8 h after drug administration. Twentyfour hours after application oxprenolol saliva concentrations were still measurable only in patient 6 (Fig. 6). Urinary excretion of oxprenolol within 36 h ranged from 0.6 to 11.8 mg in four patients. The excretion was highest during the period from 12−24 h (Fig. 7) [11].

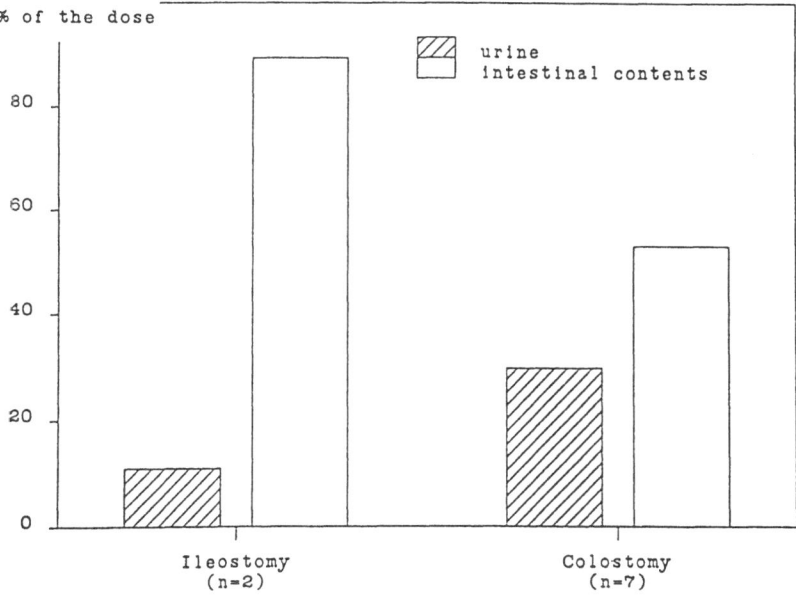

Fig. 5
Cumulative amount of clioquinol after oral administration in urine and intestinal contents of patients with stoma.

47

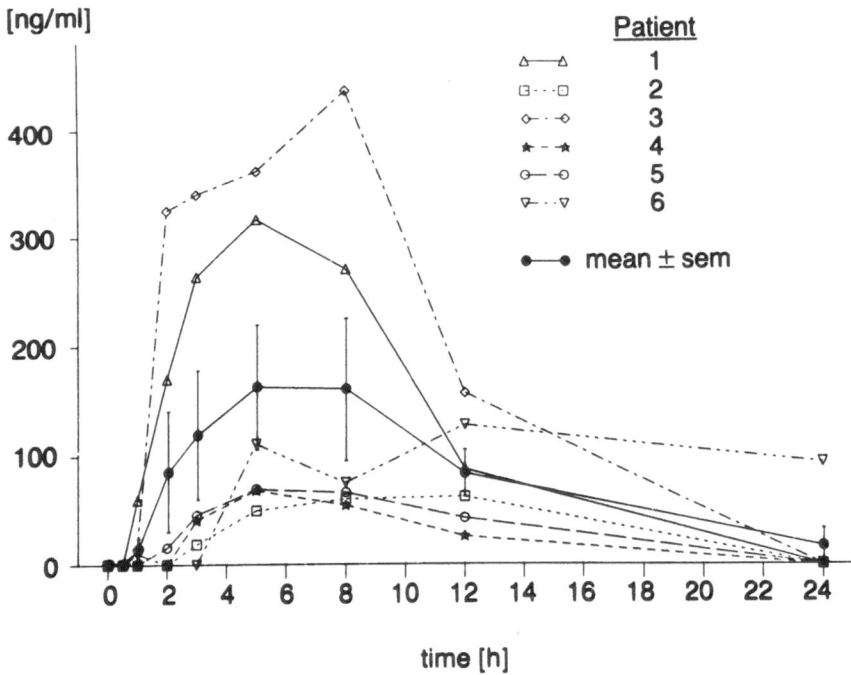

Fig. 6
Oxprenolol saliva concentrations after intrastoma application of one oxprenolol OROS®.

Discussion

The techniques employed in studying absorption in the large intestine have been reviewed recently [9, 1]. So far colonic drug absorption in man has been measured in only in a few studies [9].

In order to evaluate the absorptive capacity of the colonic mucosa we used colonoscopy in two studies with healthy volunteers to examine the colonic absorption of the beta-adrenergic blocker oxprenolol and the nonsteroidal anti-inflammatory drug diclofenac-Na. In two studies with patients with intestinal stomata we examined the colonic absorption of oxprenolol and clioquinol.

Since the beginning of the seventies colonoscopy has become a routine procedure in diagnosis and treatment of colonic diseases. Technical development of instruments which are easier to handle, thus providing a shorter and more acceptable procedure for patients has increased the usage of this method [17]. Dissolved drugs can be delivered under visual and fluoroscopic control through instrumental channels of the colonoscope. Colonoscopy when performed by an experienced endoscopist is a safe and quick procedure. Complications are very rare. The most dangerous (perforation and heavy bleeding) occur in less than 0.3% of cases [17], mainly in patients with a colon diseased by inflammation,

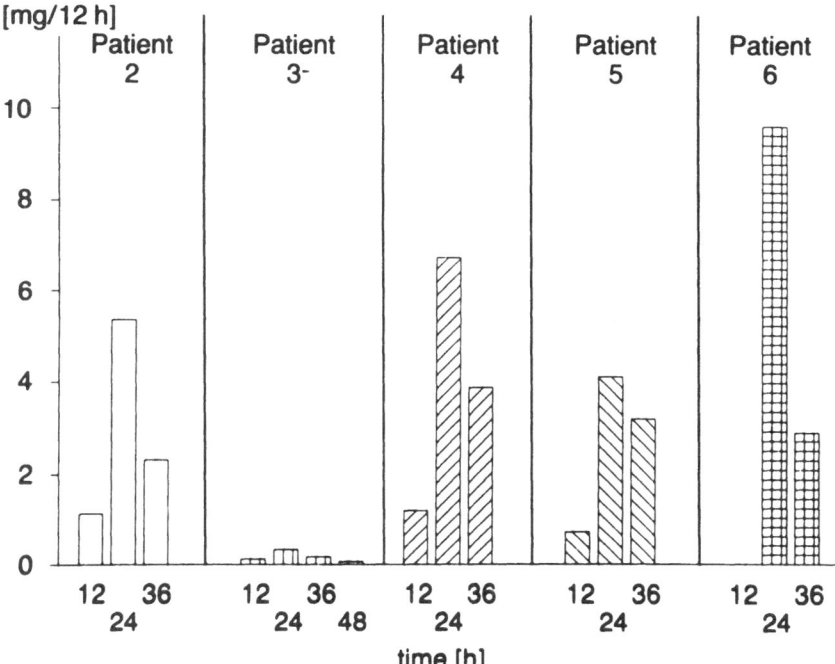

Fig. 7

Urinary excretion of oxprenolol after intrastoma application of one oxprenolol OROS®.

diverticulosis or malignoma. Respiratory problems only arise when sedatives are used. When employing colonoscopy for studying drug absorption in healthy volunteers these risks are neglegible. A well-trained endoscopist can perform a complete examination identifying the portions of the colon up to the ileocecal valve and placing the drug into distinct areas within 5 to 20 min (mean 11 min).

It should be noted that the large intestine must be well cleaned prior to endoscopy, which leads to the criticism of assessing absorption from the large bowel under non-physiological conditions. However, this holds true also for most oral bioavailability studies. In order to avoid the many non-specific effects of meals [18] absorption studies are usually performed in the fasting state. It has also been argued that laxatives given may produce superficial inflammation of the colonic mucosa thereby changing the absorptive properties. However, from clinical experience and own unpublished results it is well documented that biopsies obtained from an apparently normal colonic mucosa show also normal histological findings. Pretreatment with cleansing enemas was shown not to influence the absorption of neomycin given by enema [19]. Own studies with sulfasalazine show an absolute bioavailability of 71% for sulfapyridine absorbed from the large intestine and these subjects were not pretreated to empty the bowels [9].

The site of application (cecum or left flexure) did not influence the results. This is an interesting finding because regional differences in the absorptive capacity of the human colon concerning salt and water are well known. The ascending colon handles large volumes of ileal effluent and absorbs salt avidly. The mucosa is considered better permeable than in the descending colon which is capable of maintaining large concentration gradients generated across the mucosa [20]. The higher relative bioavailability of oxprenolol in subject 6, and of diclofenac-Na in subject 4 after administration into the left flexure could be due to colonic effluents into the rectum. Rectal absorption is known to bypass the liver [21]. The reduced hepatic first-pass-effect could explain the higher amount of drug available systemically.

Voltaren® 50 ist an enteric-coated formulation. This explains the considerable longer time to peak (t_{max}) after oral compared to colonic application of the drug.

This new indication for colonoscopy proved to be simple, is well tolerated and seems well suited for phase I studies with new compounds or new drug-formulations.

Drug absorption by the colonic mucosa can be investigated also in patients with intestinal stomata if no stenosis is present. Intestinal stomata are often used for treatment of malignant or benign diseases of the gastrointestinal tract. They can be constructed temporarily or permanently as loop or end stoma. Stomata can be used in two ways to study drug absorption. First, intestinal content of upper parts of the gastrointestinal tract can be collected from end stomata. After oral drug intake the non-absorbed portion of the dose can be recovered via the stoma and indicates the extent of absorption between mouth and stoma. Studying patients with end stomata of different parts of the gastrointestinal tract may give hints of the place and the extent of absorption. Furthermore, for example, this method may also be valuable for getting information on effective bactericidal intracolonic concentrations after oral antimicrobial therapy or on therpeutic intracolonic drug concentration after new oral formulations of 5-amino salicylic acid.

Second, in patients with a loop stoma drugs can be introduced into the distal part. By measurement of drug concentrations in body fluids the absorptive capacity between stoma and anus can be assessed.

The results gained after application of an oxprenolol OROS® into a stoma confirm qualitatively the data obtained after intracolonic administration of oxprenolol in healthy young volunteers during colonoscopy. With both techniques it could be demonstrated that the beta-adrenoceptor antagonist oxprenolol is well absorbed by the colonic mucosa. It can be concluded: both, colonoscopy and studies in patients with artificial stomata are useful to investigate drug absorption by the colonic mucosa in man.

Colonoscopy allows the quantitative measurement of the relative colonic bioavailability of a drug. On the other hand it causes discomfort to the volunteers, needs a clean colon and radiological equipment. Colonoscopy should only be performed by a skilled endoscopist.

Investigations on patients with artifical stomata must be performed in a hospital. There is no discomfort to the patients but they can give only qualitative indications of the absorptive capacity of the part of the gastrointestinal tract investigated.

Measuring saliva concentrations of drugs in patients with stoma can prevent unnecessary blood loss.

References

[1] R. Shields: Absorption from the human colon. In: *Duthie H.L.*, Wormsley K.G., eds. Scientific basis of gastroenterology. Edinburgh, London and New York: Churchill-Livingstone, 398–414, (1979).

[2] K.H. Antonin, P.R. Bieck, Ch. Schick, B. Steidle: Vergleichende chemische und radiologische Bestimmung der intestinalen Passagezeit (PZ) (Mund/Zoekum). Z. *Gastroenterologie*, 20, 554–555, (1982).

[3] S.S. Davis, J.G. Hardy, J.W. Fara: Transit of pharmaceutical dosage forms through the small intestine. *Gut*, 27, 886–892, (1986).

[4] J.H. Cummings, H.S. Wiggins: Transit through the gut measured by analysis of a single stool. *Gut*, 17, 219–223, (1976)

[5] V.A. John, P.A. Shotton, J. Moppert, W. Theobald: Gastrointestinal transit of Oros drug delivery systems in healthy volunteers: a short report. *Br. J. Clin. Pharmac.*, 19, 203S–206S, (1985)

[6] N.W. Read, C.A. Miles, D. Fisher, A.M. Holgate, N.D. Kime, M.A. Mitchell, A.M. Reeve, T.B. Roche, M. Walker: Transit of a meal through the stomach, small intestine, and colon in normal subjects and its role in the pathogenesis of diarrhea. *Gastroenterology*, 79, 1276–1282, (1980).

[7] F. Theeuwes: Novel drug delivery systems. In Drug absorption: Proceedings of the Edinburgh International Conference, eds Prescott L.F. and Nimmo W.S. *ADIS Press*, Hong Kong, 157–176, (1981).

[8] J. Urquhart: Rate-controlled drug dosage. *Drugs*, 23, 207–222, (1982).

[9] P.R. Bieck: Arzneistoffresorption aus dem menschlichen Dickdarm – neue Erkenntnisse. *Acta Pharm. Technol.*, 33, 109–114 (1987).

[10] K.H. Antonin, P.R. Bieck, M. Scheurlen, M. Jedrychowski, H. Malchow: Oxprenolol absorption in man after single bolus dosing into two segments of the colon compared with that after oral dosing. *Br. J. Clin. Pharmacol.*, 19, 137S–142S, (1985).

[11] K.H. Antonin, U. Wiest, P.R. Bieck: Colonic absorption of oxprenolol in man delivered by an oral osmotic delivery system (OROS®). *Acta Pharmacol. Toxicol.*, 59, (Suppl. V), 86, (1986).

[12] C.H. Gleiter, C. Cremer, P. Bieck, N. Hengen, G. Kieninger, W. Schönleber: Nicht-invasive Untersuchung der Arzneistoffabsorption in verschiedenen Dünn- und Dickdarmbereichen. Z. *Gastrenterologie*, 22, 509, (1984).

[13] C.H. Gleiter, K.H. Antonin, P. Bieck, J. Godbillon, W. Schönleber, H. Malchow: Colonoscopy in the investigation of drug absorption in healthy volunteers. *Gastrointestinal Endoscopy*, 31, 71–73, (1985).

[14] P.H. Degen, W. Riess: Simplified method for the determination of oxprenolol and other beta-receptor blocking agents in biological fluids by gas-liquid chromatography. *J. Chromatogr.*, 121, 72–75, (1976).

[15] J. Godbillon, S. Gauron, J.P. Metayer: High performance liquid chromatographic determination of diclofenac and its mono-hydroxylated metabolites in biological fluids. *J. Chromatogr. Biomed. Appl.*, 338, 151–159, (1985).

[16] P.H. Degen, W. Schneider, P. Vuillard, U.P. Geiger, W. Riess: The determination of clioquinol in biological materials by extractive alkylation and gas-liquid chromatography. *J. Chromatogr.*, 117, 407–413, (1976).

[17] D.G. Colin-Jones, R. Cockel, K.F.R. Schiller: Current endoscopic practice in the United Kingdom. *Clinics in Gastroenterology*, 7, 775–786, (1978).

[18] J.P. Griffin: Drug interactions occurring during absorption from the gastrointestinal tract. *Parmac. Ther.*, 15, 79–88, (1981).

[19] K.J. Breen, R.E. Bryant, J.D. Levinson, S. Schenker: Neomycin absorption in man. Studies of oral and enema administration and effect of intestinal ulceration. *Ann. Int. Med.*, 76, 211–218, (1972).

[20] P.C. Hawker, L.A. Turnberg. In: Alexander-Williams J., Binder H.J., eds. *Large intestine*, London: Butterworths 1–15, (1983).

[21] A.G. De Boer, F. Moolenaar, L.G.J. De Leede, D.D. Breimer: Rectal drug administration: clinical pharmacokinetic considerations. *Clin. Pharmacokin.*, 7, 285–311, (1982).

Diskussion

Frage
Bestehen zwischen Probanden und Patienten bzgl. der Verallgemeinerungsfähigkeit von Untersuchungsergebnissen Unterschiede, wenn die Tatsache Berücksichtigung findet, daß an Patienten gewonnene Ergebnisse mit hoher Wahrscheinlichkeit mit pathologischen gastrointestinalen Bedingungen verbunden waren?

Antwort
In der Tat kann hier häufig nicht von normalen Verhältnissen ausgegangen werden. Das hat aber die Untersuchungsmethode an Stomaträgern mit anderen Untersuchungsmethoden gemeinsam. Allerdings wurden unsere Untersuchungen in der Regel kurz vor der Rückverlegung des Stomas durchgeführt. Röntgenologisch waren keine pathologischen Veränderungen erkennbar, woraus geschlossen werden kann, daß die Schleimhautverhältnisse bei diesen Patienten normal waren.

Theophyllin.
Absorption in verschiedenen Darmabschnitten

A.H. Staib[1], D. Loew[1], S. Harder[1], J. Kollath[2], E.H. Graul[3],
O. Schuster[4], B. Hugemann[4]

[1]Abteilung Klinische Pharmakologie, [2]Zentrum der Radiologie, Abteilung Allgemeine Radiologie; Klinikum der Johann Wolfgang Goethe-Universität, D-6000 Frankfurt 70.
[3]Institut für Environtologie und Nuklearmedizin, Klinikum der Philipps-Universität, D-3550 Marburg/Lahn.
[4]PAZ GmbH, Bereich Arzneimittelentwicklung, D-6230 Frankfurt 80.

Summary

The absorption of a theophylline solution delivered to different sites of the gastro-intestinal tract in doses between 80–120 mg has been determined in 7 male volunteers using a remote controlled drug release system (HF-capsule). Absorption measurements obtained by application of the substance with this method into the stomach was comparable to the conventional oral application of a theophylline solution as demonstrated by results with both methods in the same subject. No differences exist between the stomach, the ileum, and the colon in the amount of theophylline absorbed (AUC). The calculated $T_{1/2abs}$ of theophylline absorbed via the colon were prolonged when compared with the upper gastro-intestinal tract. Results provide a rational basis for the development of further theophylline formulations and are indispensible for the explanation of variations in bioavailability of theophylline-retard drug preparations. Therefore, the absorption characteristics of theophylline make it possible to develop sustained release products for b.i.d. dosing or less frequently.

Einleitung

Die Absorption ist ein bestimmender Faktor der Verfügbarkeit eines Arzneimittels und eine Voraussetzung für seine orale oder enterale Anwendbarkeit. Als ein typisch biologischer Vorgang muß der Absorptionsprozeß von vorangehenden oder parallel wirksamen Einflüssen auf die Bioverfügbarkeit klar abgegrenzt werden, im allgemeinen kann der Absorptionsablauf für eine bestimmte Substanz durch technische oder galenische Maßnahmen über den biologisch vorgegebenen Rahmen hinaus qualitativ nicht verändert werden.
Routineuntersuchungen zur Absorption, Verteilung und Elimination einer per os verabreichten Substanz, wie sie z.B. im Rahmen von Bioverfügbarkeits- Studien erfolgen, ergeben in der Regel zu möglichen regionalen Unterschieden der Absorption im Verlauf des Magen-Darmtraktes (GIT) keine direkt verwertbaren Daten.

Der für eine Analyse lokalisationsabhängiger Unterschiede der Absorption geringe Diskriminationswert von Studien mit einfacher oraler Substanzapplikation hat verschiedene Gründe:

1. *Absorptionsvorgänge beginnen sofort,* sofern Schleimhaut und Substanz im „absorptionsgeeigneten Zustand" vorliegen
2. *Absorption erfolgt solange, wie ein Konzentrationsgefälle* in Richtung der systemischen Zirkulation *existiert,* d.h. solange Substanz im luminalen Teil des GIT vorhanden ist
3. wegen der in der Regel verabreichten Substanzmenge und aus zeitlichen Gründen sind Absorptionsvorgänge daher auf die *oberen Abschnitte des Magen-Darmtraktes begrenzt*
4. *gleichzeitig wirksame Faktoren* (Galenik, Löslichkeit, Darminhalt usw.) *modifizieren die absorbierte Menge* durch Änderungen der Bereitstellung der Substanz, *aber nicht* den biologischen *Grundvorgang* der Penetration und den Ort der Absorption selbst.

Eine genaue Abklärung des Absorptionsverhaltens ist andererseits aber häufig von besonderem Interesse, z.B. bei Substanzen, die Dosierungsprobleme aufweisen, die langfristig wiederholt verabreicht werden sollen und bei denen galenische Optimierungen therapeutisch zweckmäßig erscheinen.

Problemstellung

Resorptionsunterschiede in verschiedenen Darmabschnitten interessieren bei dem Wirkstoff Theophyllin praktisch aus folgenden Gründen:

– optimale Entwicklung von Retardpräparationen, besonders der Ermittlung von sog. „Resorptionsfenstern"
– Einfluß pathophysiologischer Faktoren (Diarrhoe, Füllungszustand, Transit u.a.) auf die Verfügbarkeit
– Differenzierung von lokalen Nebenwirkungen.

Die methodischen Möglichkeiten der an beliebigen Stellen des GIT auslösbaren HF-Kapsel [1] haben wir in den im Folgenden dargestellten Untersuchungen genutzt, um Grundlagen zu möglichen Unterschieden der Absorptionsrate und -menge für Theophyllin am Menschen zu gewinnen.

Um bei der Studie definierte und kontrollierte Bedingungen zu sichern, sind wir von einer Studienanlage ausgegangen [2], die folgende Aussagemöglichkeiten gewährleistet:

– *sukzessiver Ausschluß* proximal vom Auslösungsort gelegener *Absorptionsanteile*
  = *enge Staffelung* der Freigabelokalisationen, besonders in den tieferen GIT-Abschnitten;
– Einbeziehung einer gastralen Freigabe zum Vergleich mit der oralen Applikation
  = *Nachweis der Freigabevollständigkeit* aus der HF-Kapsel;
– Applikation in einer *Zubereitungsform*, die galenische Einflüsse auf den Absorptions-Zeitverlauf möglichst ausschließt,
  = Anwendung einer *Lösung*;
– *Standardisierung* der physiologischen und kinetischen Bedingungen, um die Vergleichbarkeit der Ergebnisse kontinuierlich zu sichern,
  = *intraindividueller Vergleich*; Nachweis konstanter Eliminationsparameter.

Material und Methoden

Wir haben mit dieser Methode die Absorption von Theophyllin im intraindividuellen Vergleich bei insgesamt sieben männlichen Erwachsenen in den Jahren 1985–1987 untersucht (Tabelle 1).

Folgende Freigabelokalisationen bzw. Theophyllinapplikationen wurden bei den Versuchspersonen realisiert:

orale Applikation einer Lösung, HF-Kapsel-Freigabe im Magen, im terminalen Ileum und in drei verschiedenen Colonabschnitten (Colon ascendens, transversum/ descendens und sigmoideus) (Abb. 1).

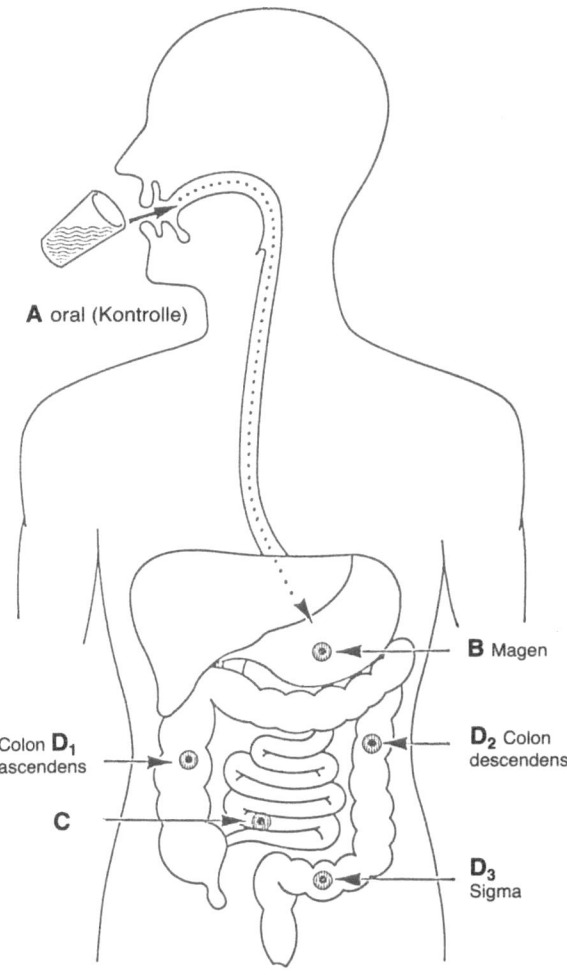

Abb. 1
Lokalisationen der Theophyllinfreisetzung und Bezeichnungen.

Die Versuchspersonen erhielten morgens nüchtern nach einem methylxanthinfreien 24-Stunden-Intervall eine Solldosis von 100 mg Theophyllin in Form einer handelsüblichen Theophyllinlösung (mit Natriumsalicylamid als Lösungsvermittler). Diese wurde entweder im Arzneireservoir der HF-Kapsel oder per os mit etwa 250 ml Mineralwasser appliziert[1].

Tabelle 1.

Personendaten:			*Untersuchungsgruppen:*					
code	Alter[1)	KG (kg)	A	B	C	D_1	D_2	D_3
1	27	85	*	*	2·*	*	**	**
2	48	82	*	*	2·*	**	**	*
3	50	74	*	*	*	**	*	**
4	26	75	**	–	2·**	**	?	**
5	23	64	2·**	–	**	**	**	**
6	26	62	**	–	**	?	?	**
7	28	71	**	–	**	**	?	**

Untersuchungstermine:						
Kontrolle		HF-Freisetzung in:				
code	A	B	C	D^1	D^2	D^3
1	15.02.85	28.06.85	17.04.85 13.05.85	09.07.86	31.05.85	17.07.86
2	15.02.85	13.05.85 17.04.85	31.05.85	09.07.86	28.08.86	28.06.85
3	15.02.85	13.03.85	17.04.85	28.06.85	31.05.85	09.03.86
4	04.07.86		09.07.86	28.08.86	05.08.86?	17.07.86 03.12.86
5	04.07.86 03.12.86		13.08.86	28.08.86	09.07.86	05.08.86
6	28.07.86		17.07.86	28.08.86?	13.08.86?	05.08.86
7	17.12.86		03.12.86	10.12.86	27.01.87?	14.01.87

[1) zu Studienbeginn;
* = Studie I (Untersuchung 1985); Eur. J. Clin. Pharmacol. 30,691−697 (1986);
** = Studie II;
− = keine Untersuchung;
? = Ergebnis aus technischen Gründen nicht auswertbar, in Folgetabellen mit (−) bezeichnet;
2· = zweimalige Untersuchung der gleichen Lokalisation

---

1 aus technischen Gründen konnte nicht bei allen Freiwilligen der gesamte Untersuchungszyklus realisiert werden (s. Tabelle 1).

Die Lokalisation des Arzneiträgers wurde vor der Freisetzung des Theophyllins röntgenologisch dokumentiert und die Auslösung durch eine Nachkontrolle (Position der Auslöse-Nadel) überprüft und gesichert.

Nach der Freisetzung wurde der Verlauf der Theophyllin-Plasmakonzentrationen in venös entnommenen Blutproben über 24 Stunden verfolgt. Die Theophyllinbestimmung erfolgte mittels HPLC [3].

Als Parameter zur Beurteilung der Absorption dienten die Fläche unter der Plasmakonzentrationszeitkurve (AUC) und die Absorptionshalbwertszeit ($T_{1/2abs}$); weiterhin wurden C_{max}, T_{max}, die mittlere Verweildauer (MT) sowie die Eliminationshalbwertszeit ($T_{1/2el}$) ermittelt. Die Berechnung der Werte erfolgte durch zwei Arbeitsgruppen mit verschiedenen voneinander unabhängigen Verfahren [2].

Ergebnisse

Der *Verlauf der Konzentrationswerte* soll in den folgenden Beispielen, die einerseits die Vergleichbarkeit der Applikationsmethode HF-Kapsel mit konventionellen Methoden und andererseits den intraindividuellen Ablauf veranschaulichen, dargestellt werden:

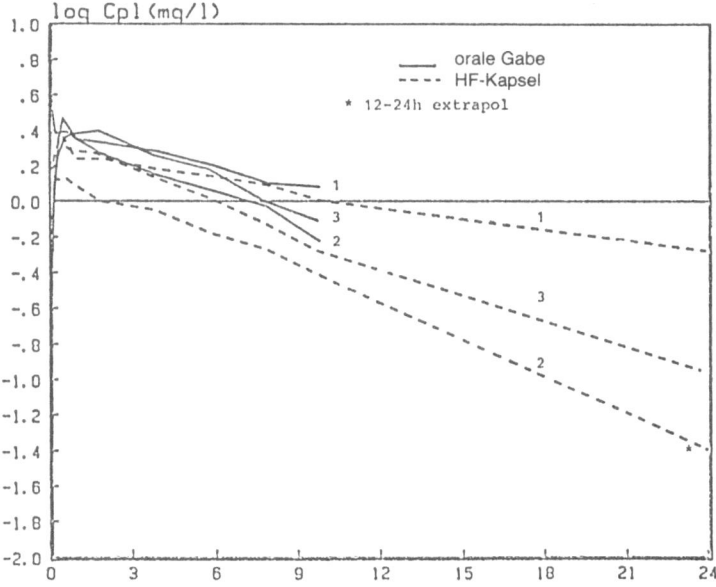

Abb. 2
Konzentrations-Zeit-Verläufe orale Gabe versus HF-Magen für drei Versuchspersonen.

Abb. 2 zeigt intraindividuell am Beispiel von drei Versuchspersonen den Vergleich einer oralen Applikation und einer Substanzfreisetzung im Magen; unter Berücksichtigung der etwas unterschiedlichen Dosierungen zeigen sich übereinstimmende Kurvenverläufe, damit ist die Vergleichbarkeit der Ergebnisse u.E. durch übereinstimmende Verfügbarkeit und sich entsprechende Eliminationswerte bei Routinemethode (orale Applikation) und bei gastraler Freisetzung (HF-Kapsel) belegt.

Abb. 3 (Versuchsperson Nr. 3 DL) stellt den intraindividuell verglichenen Verlauf der Plasmakonzentrationen bei allen Untersuchungsdurchgängen dar.

Es ist erkennbar, daß der Kurvenverlauf mit Ausnahme der initialen Abschnitte keine wesentlichen lokalisationsabhängigen Unterschiede aufweist.

Die berechneten kinetischen Parameter (Tabellen 4–7) der Versuchspersonen unterscheiden sich zwar hinsichtlich der Eliminationsparameter interindividuell, jedoch findet sich intraindividuell (Tabelle 6, $T_{1/2el}$) zwischen den verschiedenen Freisetzungslokalisationen keine wesentliche Abweichung; gleiches zeigte sich für die AUC-Werte (Tabelle 4, AUC).

Dagegen weisen die initialen Kurvenläufe (Tabelle 5, Vergleich der $T_{1/2abs}$) auf einen Verzögerungstrend der Absorptionsgeschwindigkeit in der Reihenfolge der Freisetzungsorte

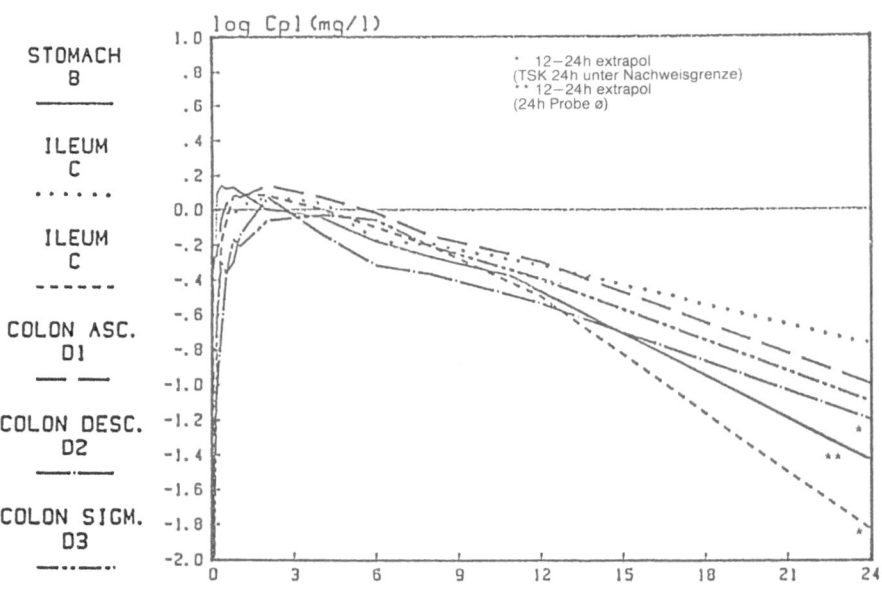

Abb. 3

Konzentrations-Zeitverläufe aller Durchgänge der Versuchsperson DL (intraindividueller Vergleich).

Magen-Ileum-Colon ascendens-Colon sigmoides hin, der sich auch in einer Zunahme der mean time-Werte (Tabelle 7) ausdrückt.

Die grafischen Darstellungen demonstrieren zusammenfassend für die AUC lokalisationsunabhängig die Vollständigkeit der Theophyllinabsorption (Abb. 4, Übereinstimmung der Mediane). Ferner wird (Abb. 5) der von oral nach caudal zunehmende Zeitbedarf für die Absorption (Zunahme der Medianwerte nach caudal) deutlich.

Tabelle 2. Maximale Plasmakonzentration (C_{max}[***], $mg \cdot l^{-1}$)

	A	B	C*; C**	D1	D2	D3
1.	2.97	2.36	1.91/1.51	2.35	1.40	2.09
2.	3.49	1.39	1.17/1.24	1.38	1.15	0.94
3.	2.53	2.11	1.78	1.35	1.41	1.44
4.	3.54	–	1.05/1.75	0.75	(–)	1.50
5.	4.07/5.59		2.16	1.17	1.82	1.06
6.	3.94	–	2.83	(–)	(–)	2.56
7.	3.54	–	2.66	1.36	(–)	2.17
Median:	3.49* (N = 11)		1.77 (N = 10)	1.36	1.41	1.50

[***] absolute Dosen in A höher als in B bis D3, keine Dosiskorrekturen; [*/**] s. Tab. 1

Tabelle 3. T_{max} (Stunden)

	A	B	C*; C**	D1	D2	D3
1.	0.5	0.5	0.75/2.0	1.0	4.0	1.0
2.	0.17	0.38	2.0/1.0	2.0	2.0	4.0
3.	2.0	0.75	1.0	2.05	2.12	2.0
4.	0.33	–	2.0/0.5	4.0	(–)	1.0
5.	0.33/0.33	–	0.5	4.0	0.33	2.0
6.	0.66	–	0.66	(–)	(–)	0.17
7.	0.5	–	0.16	2.0	(–)	0.17
Median:	0.5 (N = 11)		0.83 (N = 10)	2.0	2.1	1.0

Tabelle 4. Fläche unter der Plasmakonzentration-Zeit-Kurve (AUC, $mg \cdot h \cdot l^{-1}$)

	A	B	C*; C**	D1	D2	D3
1.	22.9	23.5	22.4/20.3	27.1	22.5	24.3
2.	12.3	10.8	12.2/11.2	10.6	9.1	9.4
3.	14.0	14.5	11.1	11.1	12.2	12.6
4.	13.9	–	8.9/9.2	9.2	(–)	11.3
5.	14.8/20.6	–	14.9	18.2	13.9	15.2
6.	14.7	–	13.6	(–)	(–)	12.7
7.	14.44	–	15.9	13.8	(–)	15.2
Median:	14.5 (N = 11)		12.9 (N = 10)	12.5	13.1	12.7

Tabelle 5. Absorptionshalbwertzeit ($T_{1/2abs}$, Stunden)

	A	B	C*; C**	D1	D2	D3
1.	0.13	0.4	0.12/0.38	0.16	0.46	0.34
2.	0.08	0.15	0.72/0.61	0.62	0.64	1.34
3.	0.29	0.14	0.14	0.45	1.49	0.99
4.	0.36	–	0.63/0.60	0.78	(–)	0.55
5.	0.1/0.1	–	0.1	1.5	0.05	1.74
6.	0.1	–	0.84	(–)	(–)	1.54
7.	0.1	–	0.13	0.45	(–)	0.97
Median:	0.13 (N = 11)		0.49 (N = 10)	0.54	0.55	0.99

Tabelle 6. Eliminationshalbwertzeit ($T_{1/2el}$, Stunden)

	A	B	C*; C**	D1	D2	D3
1.	8.6	9.2	7.3/7.6	9.62	9.2	7.45
2.	4.9	4.7	6.0/4.6	5.8	5.2	5.6
3.	5.2	5.1	4.8	5.6	4.8	5.95
4.	5.0	–	5.95/3.65	6.93	(–)	4.9
5.	4.8/7.1	–	7.52	9.96	8.36	9.1
6.	4.36	–	4.97	(–)	(–)	4.47
7.	5.8	–	5.46	6.41	(–)	7.73
Median:	5.1 (N = 11)		5.67 (N = 10)	6.7	6.8	5.95

Tabelle 7. Mittlere Verweildauer (MT, Stunden)

	A	B	C*; C**	D1	D2	D3
1.	12.6	13.4	10.6/11.6	14.2	15.3	11.2
2.	7.1	6.9	9.7/7.5	9.3	8.4	10.0
3.	7.9	7.5	7.2	8.7	9.0	10.0
4.	7.9	–	9.5/6.1	11.1	(–)	7.9
5.	7.0/10.3	–	11.0	16.5	12.1	15.6
6.	6.5	–	8.4	(–)	(–)	8.7
7.	8.5	–	8.1	9.9	(–)	12.5
Median:	7.9 (N = 11)		8.95 (N = 10)	10.5	10.6	10.0

AUC (mg*h/l)

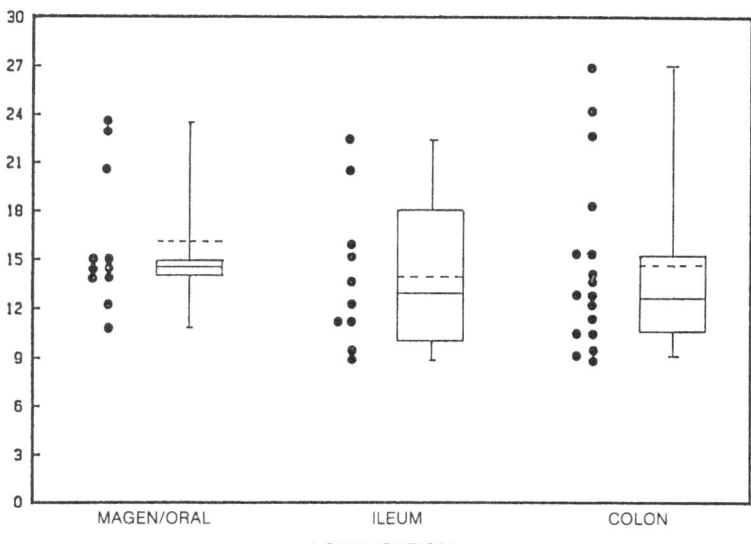

Abb. 4
Box Plot nach TUKEY: AUC.

T/2abs (h)

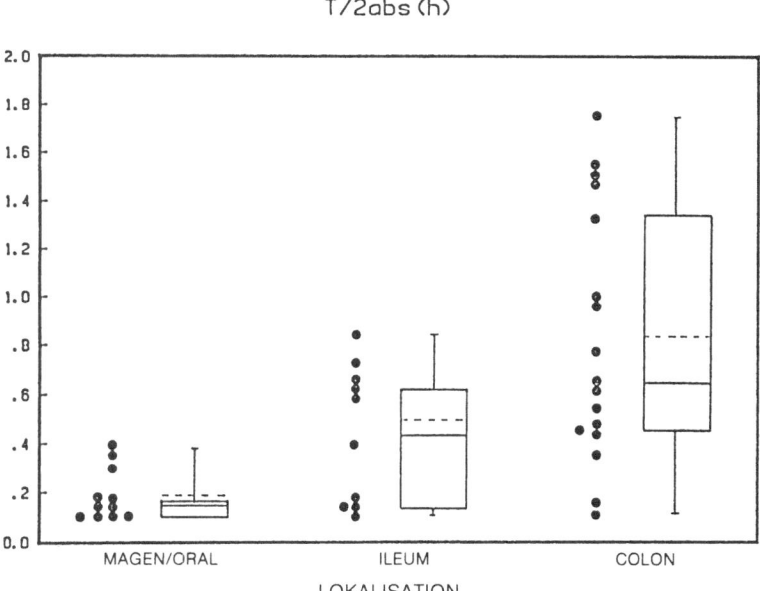

Abb. 5
Box Plot nach TUKEY: $T_{1/2abs}$.

Diskussion und Schlußfolgerungen

Die Absorptionshalbwertszeit nach oraler Applikation ist kurz (0,08 bis 0,56 Stunden), die absolute Bioverfügbarkeit einer Theophyllinlösung entspricht in den meisten Studien etwa 100%. Unsere Ergebnisse stimmen mit diesen Literaturbefunden (Übersichten bei [4–6]) überein.

Die beobachteten Differenzen der in Magen und Ileum gemessenen Werte zu den Absorptionsgeschwindigkeiten bzw. -konstanten in tieferen Darmabschnitten beruhen wahrscheinlich nicht auf Unterschieden in der Disposition, da sowohl AUC-Werte (Dost' Regel der korrespondierenden Flächen) als auch die Eliminations-Halbwertszeiten weitgehend übereinstimmten. Methodisch können wir für die unteren Colonabschnitte allerdings nicht sicher einen Einfluß von Faeces auf die Bereitstellung der freigesetzten Theophyllin-Lösung ausschließen.

Gegen einen solchen Einfluß spricht aber die auch bei Ileumfreisetzungen bereits vorhandene Veränderung der Werte. Der Mechanismus einer solchen lokalisationsabhängigen Differenz der Absorptionsgeschwindigkeit ist demnach noch nicht klar. Frühere Untersuchungen zur Theophyllinverfügbarkeit in den unteren Colon- bzw. Rektumabschnitten zeigen eine komplette Absorption rektal applizierten Theophyllins aus Klysmen und osmotischen Freisetzungssystemen [7, 8].

Unsere Ergebnisse zeigen eindeutig, daß es bei Theophyllin für den gesamten Magen-Darm-Trakt keine Hinweise auf ein „Resorptions- oder Bioverfügbarkeitsfenster" gibt. Bei Studien und in der Praxis häufig beobachtete Bioverfügbarkeitsdifferenzen bei Theophyllin-Retardpräparaten können demnach galenischen und/oder (anderen als der Resorption) physiologischen Ursachen (Füllung, Inhalt, Motilität u.ä.) zugeordnet werden.

Literatur

[1] B. Hugemann, O. Schuster: Vorrichtung zur Freisetzung von Substanzen an definierten Orten des Verdauungstraktes. Patentschrift DE 2928477 C3 (A61 K9/00) (1982).

[2] A.H. Staib, D. Loew, S. Harder, E.H. Graul, R. Pfab: Measurement of theophylline absorption from different regions of the gastro-intestinal tract using a remote controlled drug delivery device. *Eur. J. Clin. Pharmacol.* 30, 691–697 (1986).

[3] J. Caldwell, A.H. Staib, I.A. Cotgreave, M. Siebert-Weigel: Theophylline pharmacokinetics after intravenous infusion with ethylenediamine or sodium glycinate. *Br. J. clin. Pharmac.* 22, 351–355 (1986).

[4] R. Ogilvie: Clinical pharmacokinetics of theophylline. *Clin. Pharmacokin.* 3, 267–293 (1978).

[5] L. Hendeles, M. Weinberger, G. Johnson: Theophylline. In: W.E. Evans, J.J. Schentag, W.I. Jusko (eds) Applied pharmacokinetics. Principles of therapeutics drug monitoring. Applied therapeutics Inc., San Francisco, chapter 6, pp 95–138 (1980).

[6] J.G. Wagner: Estimation of theophylline absorption rate by means of the Wagner-Nelson equation. *J. Allergy Clin. Immunol.* 78(4), 2 (Suppl.), 681–688 (1986), in: Symposium Proceedings (ed. by J.A. Grant and E.F. Ellis) Update on theophylline, September 4–6, 1985 Bethesda, Maryland.

[7] P. Bolme, P.O. Edlund, M. Eriksson, L. Paalzow, B. Winbladh: Pharmacokinetics of theophylline in young children with asthma: Comparison of rectal enema and suppositories. *Eur. J. Clin. Pharmacol.* 16, 133–139 (1979).

[8] L.G.J. De Leede, A.G. De Boer, S.L. van Vuelzen, D.D. Breimer: Zero-order rectal delivery of theophylline in man with an osmotic system. *J. Pharmacokin. Biopharmac.* 10, 5, 525–537 (1982).

Indication of Absorption of Theophylline
from the Large Intestine following Administration
of Depot Preparations

B.C. Lippold
Institute of Pharmaceutical Technology, University of Düsseldorf, D-4000 Düsseldorf 1

Summary

From pharmacokinetic studies with a theophylline depot preparation it must be concluded that even in the large intestine the drug is subjected to absorption. However, absorption appears to be remarkably decelerated, while a retardation of drug liberation is also to be taken into account. Consequently plasma levels proved to decline in the terminal part of the curve more slowly. In the literature, this effect is referenced in studies with depot preparations containing other drugs and is often described as an „increase of half-life time".

Zusammenfassung

Aus pharmakokinetischen Untersuchungen mit einer Theophyllin-Depotarzneiform muß geschlossen werden, daß auch im Dickdarm noch Resorption erfolgt. Die Resorption scheint allerdings stark verlangsamt zu sein, wobei auch eine Verlangsamung der Freisetzung nicht auszuschließen ist. Insgesamt resultieren dadurch Plasmaspiegel mit abgeflachtem terminalen Bereich. Dieser Effekt wird in der Literatur auch für Depotarzneiformen mit anderen Wirkstoffen gefunden und häufig mit einer „Verlängerung der Halbwertszeit" umschrieben.

1. Introduction

On the basis of the pharmacokinetics of theophylline and a theoretical plasma level of 10 µg/ml (7.5 and 12.5 µg/ml as minimum and maximum values, respectively), a peroral depot preparation had been developed [1]. It consists of the initial dose D_i (133 mg) in the form of pellets and of the maintenance dose D_m (217 mg) in the form of microcapsules (diffusion pellets coated with ethylcellulose and polyethylene glycol 1500 as additive). The rate of release of the applied microcapsules is 22.8 + 0.8 mg/h [1, 2]. Both initial and maintenance dose are united in a hard gelatin capsule.

2. In-vivo Experiments and Evaluation

The in-vivo experiments were performed as part of an extensive cross-over study (randomized block design) in 7 healthy non-smokers. 350 mg of theophylline diluted in 70 ml water and the gelatine capsule with 70 ml were administered. The experiments were interrupted by a wash-out phase lasting 5 days. (For details see ref. [3]). Quantitative determination was performed using a ^{125}I-theophylline radioimmunoassay (Gamma-Dab^R, Travenol Comp., Munich) [4]. The calculation of pharmacokinetic parameters was provided by an analog computer [5]. A model was constructed using the constants specific to the substance administered and to volunteers obtained from the experiments following application of solutions. With the introduction of D_1 (initial dose) and D_m (maintenance dose), the following biological model was established:

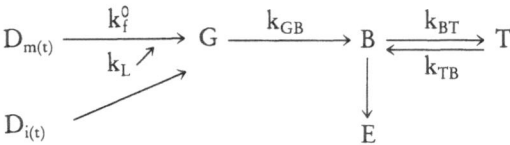

When trying to adjust the curves by mean values, a number of difficulties had to be overcome:

a) If k_f^0 and k_L are adjusted to fit the experimental points of the initial section of the data, the further course of the simulated curve no longer corresponds to the measured values (interrupted curve of mean values, Fig. 1). In all volunteers blood plasma levels between the 6th and 9th h are below the curve simulating continuous and complete liberation and absorption.

b) When trying to improve the adjustment of curves to measured data by stopping the absorption (after 7 hours the preparation enters the large intestine), part of the measured data in the terminal part (24th to 48th h) were considerably above the simulated curves (uninterrupted curve representing mean data, Fig. 1).

Thus the biological model had to be modified in order to achieve a maximum adjustment of curves on the basis of a physiologically reasonable hypothesis.

In the following it is examined how to rationalize the decreasing plasma levels after 6 to 9 hours together with continuing absorption. Several ideas may be discussed: The rate of absorption of released theophylline from the stomach and small intestine is so high that the diffusion-controlled drug liberation in that area — as planned — determines the rate of absorption. After the major part of the microcapsules has passed these areas of absorption, release is continued in the large intestine, where the drug is still absorbed, too, but at a much slower rate which is due to the reduced area of absorption and to a higher viscosity of the content. Thus absorption is rate-controlling.

As a consequence, it was necessary to reduce the rate constant of absorption in the analog computer-assisted simulation after passage of theophyllin through the stomach and small intestine, in order to take the modified conditions of absorption into account. This was done by modifying the model using the absorption rate constants for the large intestine k_{GB}' (k_a' respectively).

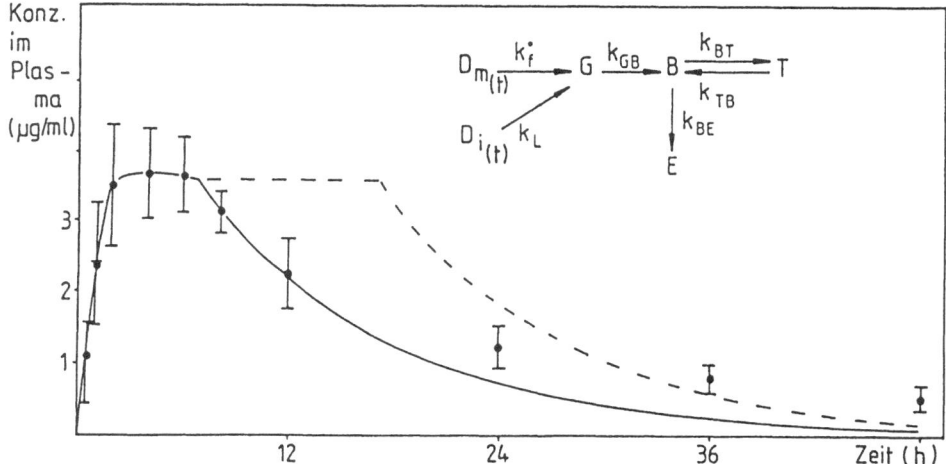

Fig. 1

Analog computer-assisted fit of plasma concentration time curves to the mean values of experimental data obtained from 7 healthy volunteers following administration of 345 mg theophylline as depot preparation ($D_i = 133$ mg; $D_m = 217$ mg)

– – – – – Simulation with continuous absorption

————— Simulation with absorption being stopped after 7 hours

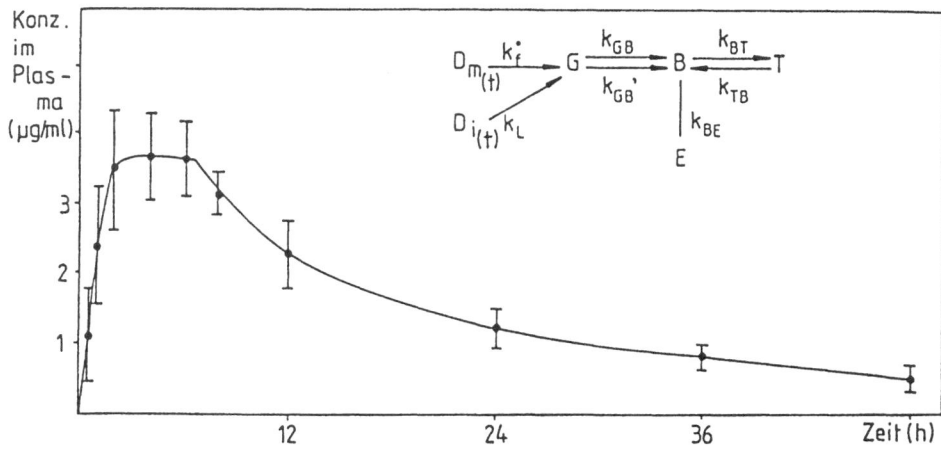

Fig. 2

Analog computer-assisted fit as in Fig. 1, but simulated deceleration of absorption rate constants after 7 hours to $k_{GB}' = 0.034$ h^{-1}.

65

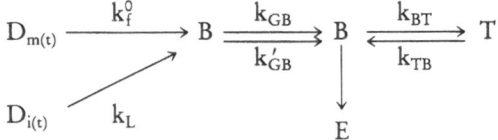

As it is shown by the fit to the mean values (Fig. 2), an excellent simulation was achieved (detailed data are given in the original paper (5)).

$$k_{GB} = 1.31 \pm 0.48 \ h^{-1} \ (t_{1/2} = 0.53 \ h),$$

$$k'_{GB} = 0.034 \pm 0.026 \ h^{-1} \ (t_{1/2} = 20.4 \ h).$$

3. References

[1] B.C. Lippold, H. Förster: *Pharm. Ind.* **44**, 735 (1982).
[2] H. Förster: *Entwicklung, Herstellung und Testung peroraler Depotarzneiformen mit konstanter Wirkstoffliberation am Beispiel des Theophyllins*, Diss. Düsseldorf (1981).
[3] G.F. Schneider, G.U. Heese, H.J. Huber, N. Janzen, H. Jünger, Ch. Moser, F. Stanislaus: *Arzneim.-Forsch./Drug Res.* 31 *(II)*, 1489 (1981).
[4] H.J. Huber, N. Janzen, G.F. Schneider, F. Stanislaus: Adaption of a commercial theophylline radioimmunoassay for use in bioavailability studies, in: *Theophylline and other Methylxanthines*, N. Rietbrock, B.G. Woodcock, A.H. Staib (Hrsg.), S. 307, Vieweg, Braunschweig (1981).
[5] B.C. Lippold, H. Förster: *Arzneim.-Forsch* **34**, 824 (1984): H. Förster, Dissertation: *Entwicklung, Herstellung und Testung peroraler Depotarzneiformen mit konstanter Wirkstoffliberation*, Düsseldorf 1981.

Diskussion

Frage
Sind die aus 3 Meßpunkten erfolgten Kurvenanpassungen aussagekräftig? Welchen Einfluß hat ferner die gefundene lange Halbwertszeit von 36 Stunden auf die Aussagekraft des Ergebnisses, wenn berücksichtigt wird, daß der langsamste Schritt der geschwindigkeits-bestimmende für Kumulationsvorgänge usw. ist? Weiterhin: Inwieweit sind in vitro gewonnene Daten mit in vivo-Daten (z.B. Dissolutionskurven mit Plasmakonzentrationszeitverläufen) vergleichbar, wenn berücksichtigt wird, daß bin in vivo ein ausschließlich der Absorption zuzuordnendes Ergebnis in der Regel kaum erreicht wird (diffusions-bedingte Einflüsse können nicht ausgeschlossen werden, Hinweis auf die Ergebnisse des Vortrags Staib und der Diskussionsbemerkung Lippold)?

Antwort
Bei Darstellung der vitro-Resultate gegen die in vivo-Ergebnisse imponiert ein biphasischer Kurvenverlauf. Dieser Verlauf entspricht genau den Zeiten, die als Transitzeiten vom Magen bis zum Dickdarm angenommen werden., Dieses Resultat ist aufgrund der Ergebnisse von Staib nur dahingehend interpretierbar, daß es sich hier ausschließlich um der Absorption zuzuordnende Vorgänge handelt, die die Grundlage des biphasischen Verlaufes wären.

Impaired Bioavailability of Theophylline Retard Preparations as a Result of pH-dependent Drug Release Rates

D. Hellenbrecht[1], C.-D. Herzfeldt[2]
Centre of Pharmacology[1], University Hospital Centre, Institute of
Pharmaceutical Technology[2], Johann Wolfgang Goethe-University,
D-6000 Frankfurt/Main 70

Summary

The galenic characterization of the release rates of Euphyllin retard — but not of
Theolair retard — showed very slow drug release at pH 5, 6, 6.8 and 7.5. This explains a number of treatment failures observed after application of Euphyllin retard
in patients with pulmonary diseases.

Non-sustained release theophylline preparations appear to be rapidly absorbed from all
sections of the intestine [1]. In sustained release preparations, however, the release can
seriously inhibit the bioavailability. This was observed in a number of patients, who were
treated with Euphyllin retard (sustained release aminophylline) because of acute aggrava-
tion of bronchial asthma or of chronic obstructive respiratory tract disease [2]. In spite
of 280 mg of a theophylline equivalent administered twice to three times daily, minimum
plasma concentration levels in 15 of those patients were below the limit of 3 mg/l, in four
patients plasma levels were too low to be detected. A dose build-up consisting of 4×1
coated tablet resulted in a mean value of 3.6 mg/l (range: $2.1-8.4$). After a change-over
to other sustained release preparations (for example 3×200 mg PulmiDur or 3×250
mg Theolair retard) theophylline plasma levels increased to about 10 mg/l.
The low degree of bioavailability of Euphyllin is obviously due to the slow rate of the
drug's release, as in 7 patients well-formed residues of the preparations were still found
in the stool. Those residues were analysed in the Central Laboratory of West-German
Pharmacists (Eschborn, FRG). It was found, that the residues still contained $70-90\%$
of active substance.
For galenic characterization of the release mechanism of Euphyllin retard, it has been
examined and compared to the reference drug Theolair retard (sustained release
theophylline) under the conditions of USP XXI [3]. The pH-values of the medium (simulated gastric juice without pepsin, simulated intestinal fluid without enzymes, and mix-
tures of the two fluids, respectively), were als follows: pH $1.2-3.0-5.0-6.0-6.8-7.5$.
These were held constant during the 12 hours test periods.
The analysis of drug release rates over the time and at different pH-values revealed that
in acid environment both preparations were released only slowly and incompletely
($60-70\%$ over 12 hours). Above pH 5.0 Theolair retard was liberated rapidly and completely within the first $6-8$ hours. Under Euphyllin as well the rate of release increased

in neutral environment. The course of Euphyllin release was biphasic, however. During the first six hours only a small fraction was liberated, and only after 6–8 hours was drug release accelerated. In contrast to the reference drug, release of Euphyllin retard was not completed in all experiments after 12 hours.

The results obtained from the drug release tests illustrate the deficient oral bioavailability of Euphyllin retard. With regard to the latest developments in technology this technique of retarding aminophyllin may be considered outdated [4].

References

[1] A.H. Staib, D. Loew, E.H. Graul, et al.: *Naunyn Schmiedebergs Arch. Pharmacol.* **330**, Suppl., R 15 (1985).
[2] D. Hellenbrecht, R. Saller, E.M. Ulmer: *Klin. Wochenschr.* **64**, Suppl. V, 219–220 (1986).
[3] C.D. Herzfeldt: *Pharm. Technol.* **8**, 70–76 (1984).
[4] R.S. Summers, B. Summers, S. Rawnsley: *Int. J. Pharm.* **30**, 83–88 (1986).

Lokalisation der Absorption von Furosemid. Befunde und Folgerungen für verschiedene Darreichungsformen

D. Loew*, A.H. Staib**, S. Harder**, O. Schuster***, E.H. Graul****

*   Fa. Medice, Kuhloweg 37-39, D-5860 Iserlohn;
**   Abtlg. Klinische Pharmakologie,
       Johann-Wolfgang-Goethe-Universität, Theodor-Stern-Kai 7, D-6000 Frankfurt/Main 70;
***   PAZ GmbH, In der Schildwacht 41, D-6230 Frankfurt/Main 80;
**** Institut für Environtologie und Nuklearmedizin,
       Philipps-Universität, Bahnhofstr. 7, D-3550 Marburg/Lahn

Summary

A prerequisite for the therapeutic effect of a drug is its sufficient bioavailability. Investigations regarding the absorption of a substance administered per os, for example, within the framework of bioavailability studies, do not generally give any information about rate and extent of the absorption in the different parts of the gastrointestinal tract (GTI) and the transit time. Such results are, however, of considerable practical interest, such as, for example, for the optimal development and judgement of retard preparations. With the remote controlled capsule (HF) the behaviour of the absorption of furosemide was investigated in the different parts of the GIT. In two studies with volunteers a decrease of the absorption from proximal to distal could be proved.

Zusammenfassung

Eine Voraussetzung für die therapeutische Wirkung eines Arzneimittels ist ihre ausreichende Bioverfügbarkeit. Untersuchungen zur Absorption einer per os verabreichten Substanz, wie sie z.B. im Rahmen von Bioverfügbarkeits-Studien erfolgen, ergeben in der Regel keine Information über Geschwindigkeit und Ausmaß der Absorption in den verschiedenen Abschnitten des Magen-Darm-Traktes und die Transitzeit. Derartige Erkenntnisse sind jedoch von erheblichem praktischen Interesse, u.a. für die optimale Entwicklung und Beurteilung von Retard-Präparaten. Mit der ferngesteuerten Arzneimittelkapsel wurde das Absorptionsverhalten von Furosemid in verschiedenen Abschnitten des Magen-Darm-Traktes untersucht. In zwei Studien an gesunden Probanden konnte ein Abfall der Absorption von proximal nach distal nachgewiesen werden.

Einleitung

Furosemid ist gegenüber den Thiaziden stärker saluretisch und diuretisch wirksam, besitzt eine günstigere Dosis-Wirkungs-Beziehung, beeinflußt nicht die glomeruläre Filtrationsrate (GFR) und verbessert die Nierendurchblutung. Trotz dieser Vorteile hat sich Furosemid in der Dauertherapie der Hypertonie bisher nicht durchgesetzt, sondern ist bislang nur hypertensiven Patienten mit eingeschränkter Nierenfunktion vorbehalten. Ursache ist die initial starke und kurze Wirkdauer von Furosemid, die zu einer Stimulation gegenregulatorischer Mechanismen führt und damit die Blutdrucksenkung abschwächt [1−4]. Um dennoch die Vorteile von Furosemid ausnutzen zu können, bot sich die Entwicklung einer galenischen Darreichungsform mit einer abgeschwächten und längeren Wirkdauer an. Als Lösungsansatz kamen Retardpellets infrage, aus denen Furosemid verzögert freigesetzt wird und damit die Substanz für eine kontinuierliche Resorption zur Verfügung steht. Wie aus in vitro-Untersuchungen (Abb. 1) hervorgeht, konnte das Problem galenisch gelöst werden [5]. Retardpräparate sind aber nur dann sinnvoll, wenn sie auch ausreichend in den tieferen Darmabschnitten absorbiert werden. Ausmaß und Geschwindigkeit der Absorption aus den verschiedenen Bereichen des Gastrointestinaltraktes lassen sich aber nur dann bestimmen, wenn die Substanz an definierten Stellen appliziert wird. Mit der ferngesteuerten Arzneimittelkapsel sind derartige Untersuchungen möglich [6]. Mit dieser Methode haben wir in zwei Probandenstudien das Absorptionsverhalten von Furosemid in verschiedenen Abschnitten des Magen-Darm-Traktes untersucht.

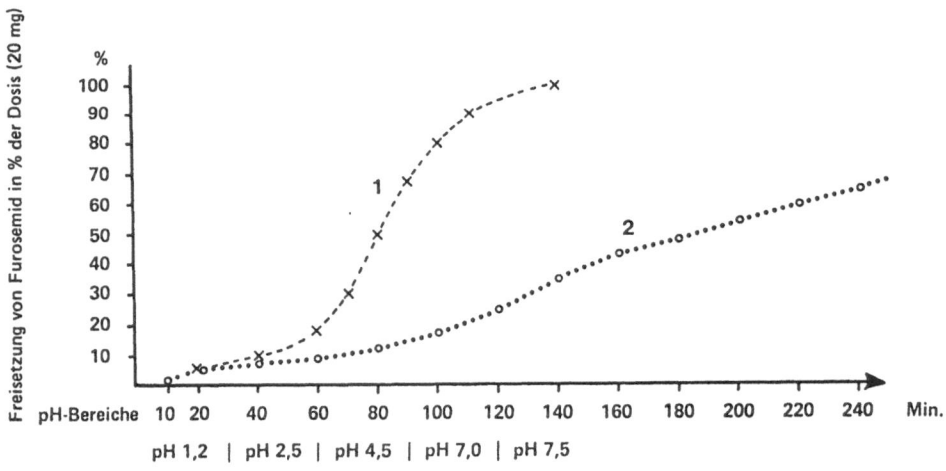

Abb. 1

In-vitro-Freisetzung von Furosemid (1) und Furosemid retard (2) in Wasser bei verschiedenen pH-Werten (nach Schulte) (10)

Methoden

Die Untersuchungen wurden an 7 männlichen Probanden im Alter von 27 bis 51 Jahren durchgeführt.

In einer interindividuellen Studie erhielten 4 Probanden nach einem Standardfrühstück zunächst 40 mg Furosemid in einer Hartgelatinekapsel und 8 Tage später unter den gleichen Versuchsbedingungen 40 mg Furosemid in der HF-Kapsel [7]. Bei 2 Probanden erfolgte die Freisetzung im Ileum und bei 2 Personen im Colon.

In einer weiteren intraindividuellen Studie erhielten 3 Probanden zunächst 40 mg Furosemid in Form einer Suspension oral. Im nächsten Untersuchungsgang wurden 40 mg Furosemid bei allen 3 Probanden mit der HF-Kapsel im Magen und dann bei einem Probanden im Jejunum und Ileum und bei 2 Probanden im Ileum und Colon freigesetzt (Abb. 2a, b).

Die Bestimmung von Furosemid erfolgte mit HPLC [8]. Die untere Nachweisgrenze im Plasma beträgt 2 ng/ml. Aus den Konzentrations-Zeitverläufen wurde die AUC nach der Trapezregel berechnet und die Absorptionsrate aus der in den jeweiligen Untersuchungsabschnitten erhaltenen und auf die Kontrolle bezogenen Werte ermittelt.

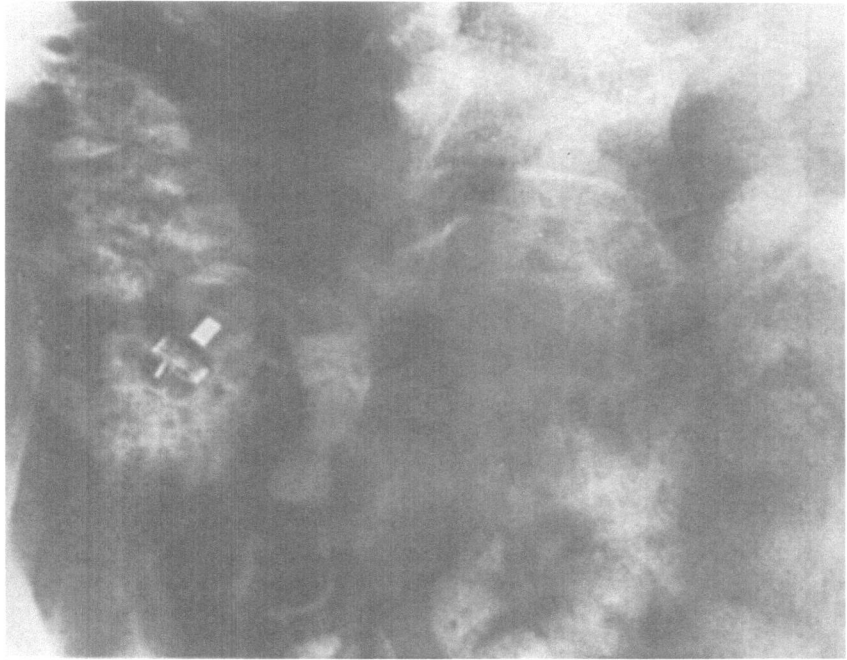

Abb. 2a

Die mit Furosemid gefüllte ungeöffnete Kapsel befindet sich am Übergang vom Ileum zum Colon (Valvula Bauhini).

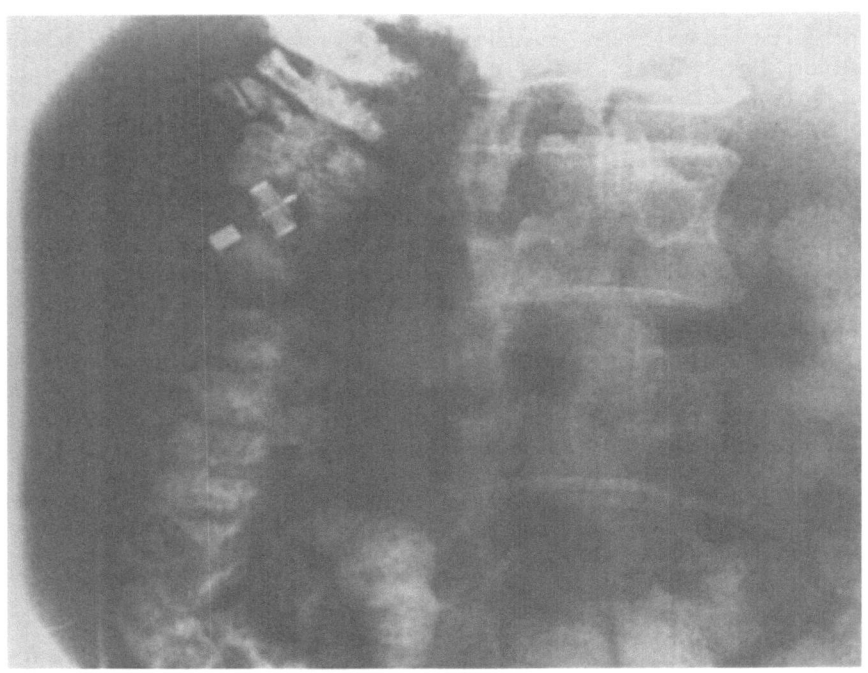

Abb. 2b
Unmittelbar nach Freisetzung von Furosemid befindet sich die HF-Kapsel im Colon ascendenz.

Ergebnisse

In Tabelle 1 sind die Ergebnisse der interindividuellen Untersuchungen mit Furosemid zusammengefaßt. Bezogen auf die Kontrolle beträgt die Absorptionsrate im Ileum 23–26% und im Colon 2,0–13,4%.

Tabelle 1. Studie I, AUC-Werte von Furosemid (ng · h · ml^{-1}) (Dosisnormierung auf 0,5 mg/kg)

Proband	Kontrolle* (100%)	HF-Freisetzung Ileum	Colon
1	1 571	409 (26.0%)	–
2	2 008	462 (23.0 %)	–
3	1 668	–	33 (2.0 %)
4	654	–	87 (13.4 %)
* orale Applikation ohne HF-Kapsel			

Die entsprechenden AUC-Werte von Furosemid in der intraindividuellen Studie sind aus Tabelle 2 zu ersehen. Hieraus ist zu erkennen, daß sich die AUC-Werte nach oraler Verabreichung von Furosemid bzw. Freisetzung aus der HF-Kapsel im Magen nur geringfügig unterscheiden. Auch im oberen Jejunum werden noch annähernd die gleichen Werte erreicht wie im Magen. Zum Ileum hin kommt es zu einem deutlichen Abfall. Hier liegen die Werte zwischen 5,1% und 24,8%. Im Colon ist nach den vorliegenden Untersuchungen praktisch keine Resorption mehr zu erwarten.

Tabelle 2. Studie II, AUC-Werte von Furosemid (ng · h · ml^{-1}) (Dosisnormierung auf 0,5 mg/kg)

Proband	Kontrolle* (100%)	Magen	HF-Freisetzung Jejunum	Ileum	Colon
1	2758	2446 (88.7%)	2392 (86.7%)	140 (5.1%)	–
2	2521	2076 (82.0%)	–	429 (17.0%)	62 (2.5%)
3	2188	1649 (75.4%)	–	543 (24.8%)	<10 (**)

* orale Applikation ohne HF-Kapsel
** Furosemid-Konzentration unterhalb der Nachweisgrenze

Diskussion und Schlußfolgerungen

In 2 Studien wurde die Absorption von Furosemid im Magen, Jejunum, Ileum und Colon untersucht. In beiden Projekten konnte übereinstimmend ein Abfall der Absorption im Gastrointestinal-Trakt von proximal nach distal nachgewiesen werden. Bei Applikation von Furosemid im Magen und Jejunum unterscheiden sich die AUC-Werte kaum voneinander. Wird jedoch Furosemid im Ileum freigesetzt, so beträgt die Resorptionsquote im Durchschnitt noch ca. 20%, während nach Applikation von Furosemid in das Colon praktisch keine Absorption mehr nachzuweisen ist.

Demgegenüber gibt es eine Reihe von Substanzen wie Isosorbid-5-Mononitrat [9], Metoprolol [10] und Theophyllin [11], die in allen Bereichen des Magen-Darm-Traktes gut absorbiert werden.

Es stellt sich nun die Frage nach den Ursachen für dieses Absorptionsverhalten. Einfluß auf die Absorption können vom Arzneimittel oder vom Absorptionsort ausgehen. Da Furosemid gesunden Probanden in einer frischen Suspension verabreicht wurde, scheiden daher primär galenische Faktoren, Interaktionen mit Medikamenten sowie Störungen der Absorption infolge Erkrankungen des Magen-Darm-Traktes aus. Für die unterschiedliche Absorption von Furosemid im Magen-Darm-Trakt können vorerst nur besondere, stoffbedingte Ursachen diskutiert werden. Hierbei bietet sich folgende Erklärungshypothese an.

Die physikalisch-chemischen Eigenschaften von Furosemid legen nach Auflösung eine komplette Absorption nahe, denn die Lipophilie der Substanz bietet unter der Voraussetzung genügend hoher Lösungsgeschwindigkeit im Darmlumen günstige Bedingungen für eine Permeation durch biologische Membranen. Aufgrund von 2 pK-Werten (3,9 und

7,5) kann selbst unter stark variierenden pH-Werten im Darmlumen immer von einem genügenden Angebot sowohl von dissoziiertem als auch undissoziiertem Anteil ausgegangen werden. Zusätzlich muß berücksichtigt werden, daß vor Übertritt in die Darmmukosa die Bereitstellungsbedingungen durch Änderung der Dissoziation noch einmal variiert wird, weil hier vermutlich niedrigere pH-Werte vorliegen als im Darmlumen. Im Dünndarm ist davon auszugehen, daß von proximal nach distal kontinuierliche pH-Verhältnisse im Lumen und an der Mukosaoberfläche vorliegen, weshalb nicht mit einer Abnahme der Absorption zu rechnen ist. Auch die Abnahme der zur Verfügung stehenden Oberfläche kann bei der gegebenen Dosis nicht als limitierender Faktor für die Absorptionsminderung angesehen werden. Für die Interpretation der Befunde kommen letztlich nur noch lokalisationstypische Veränderungen der biologischen Membran oder Probleme der Löslichkeit von Furosemid in Frage. Da ein Furosemid-spezifisches Membranverhalten (Carrier-Mechanismus) mit Abnahme der Permeation nach distal bisher nicht beschrieben und unwahrscheinlich ist, ist zu vermuten, daß die Abnahme des erforderlichen Lösungsvolumens entlang des Intestinums der kritische Faktor für die Auflösung der als Suspension gegebenen Substanz ist. Bei lipophilen Stoffen wie Furosemid wird die Auflösung durch hohe Flüssigkeitsströme sowie durch Lösungs-begünstigende Einflüsse wie Galle, Pankreas-Sekret, Motilität verbessert. Die Tagesflüssigkeitsströme liegen bei ca. 6–10 l im oberen Duodenum, ca. 1,5–2 l im Jejunum, 0,7–1,2 l im terminalen Ileum und nur 0,1 l am Ende des Colon [12]. Die scheinbar verminderte Absorption von Furosemid in den distalen Darmabschnitten ist deshalb eigentlich keine Absorptionshemmung, sondern lediglich Ausdruck einer verminderten Bereitstellung infolge zu geringen Lösungsvolumens.

Nach unseren bisherigen Erfahrungen ist die HF-Kapsel eine geeignete Untersuchungsmethode, um Hinweise darauf zu erhalten, wo eine Absorption von Substanzen stattfindet oder ob sogenannte Absorptionsfenster gleich welcher Ursachen im Gastrointestinal-Trakt bestehen. Aus den Untersuchungen geht weiter hervor, daß bei normalen Transitzeiten eine Retardierung nur sinnvoll ist, wenn die Gesamtfreisetzung innerhalb von 6–8 Stunden erfolgt.

Literatur

[1] T.C. Brown, J.O. Davis, C.I. Jonston: Acute response in plasma renin and aldosterone secretion to diuretic. *Am. J. Physiol.* **211**, 437–441 (1966).

[2] J. Greven, O. Heidenreich: Dieueretic drugs in hypertension. In: *Handbook of Hypertension*, Vol. 3: Pharmacology of antihypertensive drugs. Hrsg.: P.A. van Zwieten, Elsevier-Verlag, New York–Amsterdam, Oxford, 66–101 (1984).

[3] F. Gross, H. Brunner, M. Ziegler: Renin-angiotensin system, aldosterone, and sodium balance. *Res. Prog. Hormone Res.* **21**, 119–177 (1965).

[4] R.A. Kelly, C.S. Wilcox, W.E. Mitch, T.W. Meyer, P.F. Souney, C.M. Rayment, P.A. Friedman, S.L. Swartz: *Response of the kidney to furosemide.* II. Effect of captopril on sodium balance. Kidney Internat. **24**, 233–239 (1983).

[5] K.E. Schulte: Pharmazeutische und galenische Gesichtspunkte für die Entwicklung eines Diuretikums. In: Workshop „*Diuretika 84*", Hrsg.: E.H. Graul, D. Loew, Bad Nauheim (1984).

[6] B. Hugemann, et al.: Deutsche Patentschrift DE 2928477 C3, (1982).

[7] E.H. Graul, D. Loew, O. Schuster: Voraussetzung für die Entwicklung einer sinnvollen Retard- und Diuretika-Kombination. *Therapiewoche* 35/38, 4277–4291 (1985).

[8] D. Loew, D. Barkow, O. Schuster, H.E. Knoell: Pharmacokinetic and pharmacodynamic study of the combination of furosemide retard and triamterene. *Eur. J. Clin. Pharmacol.* **26**, 191–195 (1984).

[9] A. Wildfeuer, H. Laufen, R. Dölling, G. Pfaff, B. Hugemann, H.E. Knoell, O. Schuster: Bedeutung galenischer Formen für die orale Therapie mit antianginösen Substanzen. *Therapiewoche* **36**,
2996−3002 (1986).
[10] U. Jonsson, et al.: *Gastrointestinal Absorption of Metoprolol in Man and Dog.* II. World Conference on Clinical, Pharmacology and Therapeutics, Rockville Pike, Bethesda, USA (1983).,
[11] A.H. Staib, D. Loew, S. Harder, E.H. Graul, R. Pfab: Measurement of theophylline absorption
from different regions of the gastro-Intestinal-tract using a remote controlled drug delivery device.
Eur. J. Clin. Pharmacol. **30**, 691−697 (1986).
[12] J. Hirtz: The gastrointestinal absorption of drugs in man: a review of current concepts and
methods of investigation. *Br. J. clin. Pharmac.* **19**, 77S−83S (1985).

Absorption of Isosorbide-5-Nitrate from the Gastrointestinal Tract

H. Laufen, A. Wildfeuer

Fa. Heinrich Mack Nachf., Abt. Pharmakologie
D-7918 Illertissen

Summary

The absorption of the antianginal drug isosorbide-5-nitrate (IS-5-N) from different regions of the gastrointestinal tract was investigated in nine male human subjects using the High Frequency-capsule (HF-capsule) technique. The HF-capsule, loaded with 20 mg IS-5-N, was opened in the stomach, duodenum, middle jejunum, and colon ascendens of two subjects each, and in the upper jejunum of another subject.

Residence times of the capsule in the gastrointestinal tract from ingestion until opening ranged from 1.1 to 2.3 hours. The absorption of IS-5-N was estimated on the basis of its plasma concentrations. Areas under the curve, peak times and peak heights proved to be not dependent on the gastrointestinal site of absorption. In most cases the absorption was completed within 30—40 min after opening of the HF-capsule.

The results suggest to reject the assumption of a local absorption window above the colon transversum. These findings could be successfully applied to the rational design of a sustained release formulation of IS-5-N.

One of the basic problems in the development of sustained release drug formulations is to reconcile the time-course of drug release with the absorption capacity of the gastrointestinal regions. Study of the drug absorption at gastrointestinal sites therefore plays a key role for the rational design of the release pattern of such formulations.

Within the scope of the development of an oral sustained release form the gastrointestinal absorption of the antianginal drug isosorbide-5-nitrate (IS-5-N) was investigated in man using a remote controlled drug release system, the High Frequency-capsule (HF-capsule). IS-5-N is a highly water-soluble neutral substance. Administered orally in solution, it is rapidly and completely absorbed without first pass removal. The half-life of elimination from plasma is in the order of 4 hours.

In previous investigations with healthy subjects oral IS-5-N formulations were examined in which the release rate was varied stepwise from very high to very low. By comparing the time curves of IS-5-N in vitro release and plasma concentrations the results of these trials could be concluded that during the first 3—5 hours after the administration absorption occured rapidly, with absorption rate constants $> 1\ h^{-1}$, and that between 5—10 hours the absorption rate slowly decreased. Drug liberated in vitro after 7—10 hours apparently was not completely absorbed. If absorption was time dependent over the first 10 hours, the existence of a local absorption window was to be considered. To investigate this, the more direct technique of the HF-capsule was employed in a trial with nine healthy volunteers. Table 1 gives details of the clinical part of the study.

The HF-capsule was loaded with an aqueous solution of 20 mg IS-5-N. In two subjects each the capsule was opened in the stomach, the duodenum, the middle jejunum and the colon ascendens, in one volunteer in the upper jejunum. Residence times of the capsule in the stomach were 1.1 h and 1.7 h, transit times ranged from 0.6 h (mouth to duodenum) and 2.3 h (mouth to colon). The IS-5-N plasma concentrations were estimated using a gas chromatographic method. Basic pharmacokinetic parameters are listed in Table 2.

Since individual plasma clearances were not known, the absorbed amounts can be discussed only approximately on the basis of the AUCs. AUCs ranged between 1360 and 2223 h × ng/ml giving no indication for a lack of absorption in any of the examined gastrointestinal regions. There seemed to be no correlation between AUCs and the sites of drug liberation. The coefficient of variation in AUC amounted to ± 15%, which was in the normal range of interindividual variation after oral IS-5-N.

Figure 1 shows the absorption time-curves of IS-5-N calculated from the plasma curves by the method of Wagner and Nelson. In the majority of cases the absorption was practically completed 30—40 min after the capsule was opened. In the subjects 4 and 8 the curves are characterized by an absorption pause between 20 and 60 min after opening the capsule. This is reflected by the comparatively late occurence of the plasma peaks in both subjects (see Table 2). Subject 4 showed the lowest measured AUC, while in subject 8 a medium AUC value was obtained, so it is not clear, whether this absorption break is connected with a reduced amount of totally absorbed drug. Anyway it has to be considered that about 50% of the totally absorbed dose in these cases were not released or absorbed at the intestinal site where the capsule was opened, but in deeper regions of the intestines.

Table 1. Absorption of IS-5-N in the gastrointestinal tract using the HF-capsule. Clinical study: 9 healthy male volunteers (61 – 95 kg body weight; age 18 – 40 y). Ingestion of the capsule with 100 ml water in morning in fasting state. Standard breakfast 1.2 – 3.0 h after administration. Blood sampling: before and 10, 20, 30, 45, 60, 90, 120, 180, 240, 360, 480, 600 min and 24 h after opening of the capsule (nominal times).

Subject No.	Site of capsule opening	Residence time of the capsule in the GI-tract until opening [h]
1	Colon ascendens	2.3
2	Duodenum	1.1
3	Colon ascendens	2.3
4	Duodenum	0.6
5	Stomach	1.1
6	Stomach	1.7
7	Jejunum (middle)	1.0
8	Jejunum (upper)	1.1
9	Jejunum (middle)	0.7

Table 2. Absorption of IS-5-N in the gastrointestinal tract.
Pharmacokinetic parameters for IS-5-N plasma concentration time-curves.

Subject No.	Site of capsule opening	AUC* [hxng/ml]	Peak concentration* [ng/ml]	Peak time [h]	Half-life of elimination [h]
5	Stomach	1691	353	0.50	2.78
6	Stomach	1947	342	0.33	3.65
2	Duodenum	1538	282	0.25	3.26
4	Duodenum	1360	182	2.00	4.04
8	Jejunum (upper)	1746	244	1.67	4.45
7	Jejunum (middle)	2008	397	0.28	3.71
9	Jejunum (middle)	2028	312	0.50	4.25
1	Colon ascendens	1678	267	0.75	4.00
3	Colon ascendens	2223	450	0.75	3.35
x̄		1802	314	0.50**	3.72
SD		271	82		0.53
CV %		15.0	26.0		14.2

* normalized t the mean body weight (78 kg)
** median

In summary, this investigation gives no indication of an absence of or even markedly reduced, absorption of IS-5-N from the examined parts of the gastrointestinal tract. Indeed the results suggest that absorption is comparable at all these sites. In any case the assumption of a local absorption window of limited size above the colon transversum has to be rejected.

The passage times of the HF-capsule to jejunum and colon observed in this trial are short compared to most transit times of single and multiple galenic units reported in the literature. This may be due to the fact, that in this experiment the assignment of subjects to sites of drug delivery occurred ad hoc and not in a randomized schedule, in order to minimize the number of x-ray controls. Transit times of drug formulation units from the pylorus to the caecum were reported to be in the order of 3−4.5 h [1, 2, 3]. In contrast to residence times in the stomach, transit times through the small intestines seem little influenced by the size and the type of the formulation unit or by the amount and nature of food taken with the drug [4, 5]. The investigations of Davis et al. and Wilson et al. have shown that single unit dosage forms such as matrix tablets and osmotic devices on administration with a light breakfast had a mean residence time in the stomach of about 3 h.

Based on these gastrointestinal transit times we made the assumption that for a sustained release tablet of IS-5-N, taken with a light breakfast, a mean period of at least 5−6 h exists, during which the absorption of the drug will not be limited by the absorptive capacity of the passed gastrointestinal regions. This assumption agrees well with the suggestion from the earlier mentioned trial with IS-5-N sustained release forms where incomplete absorption only occured when drug was released later than 7 hours after the administration.

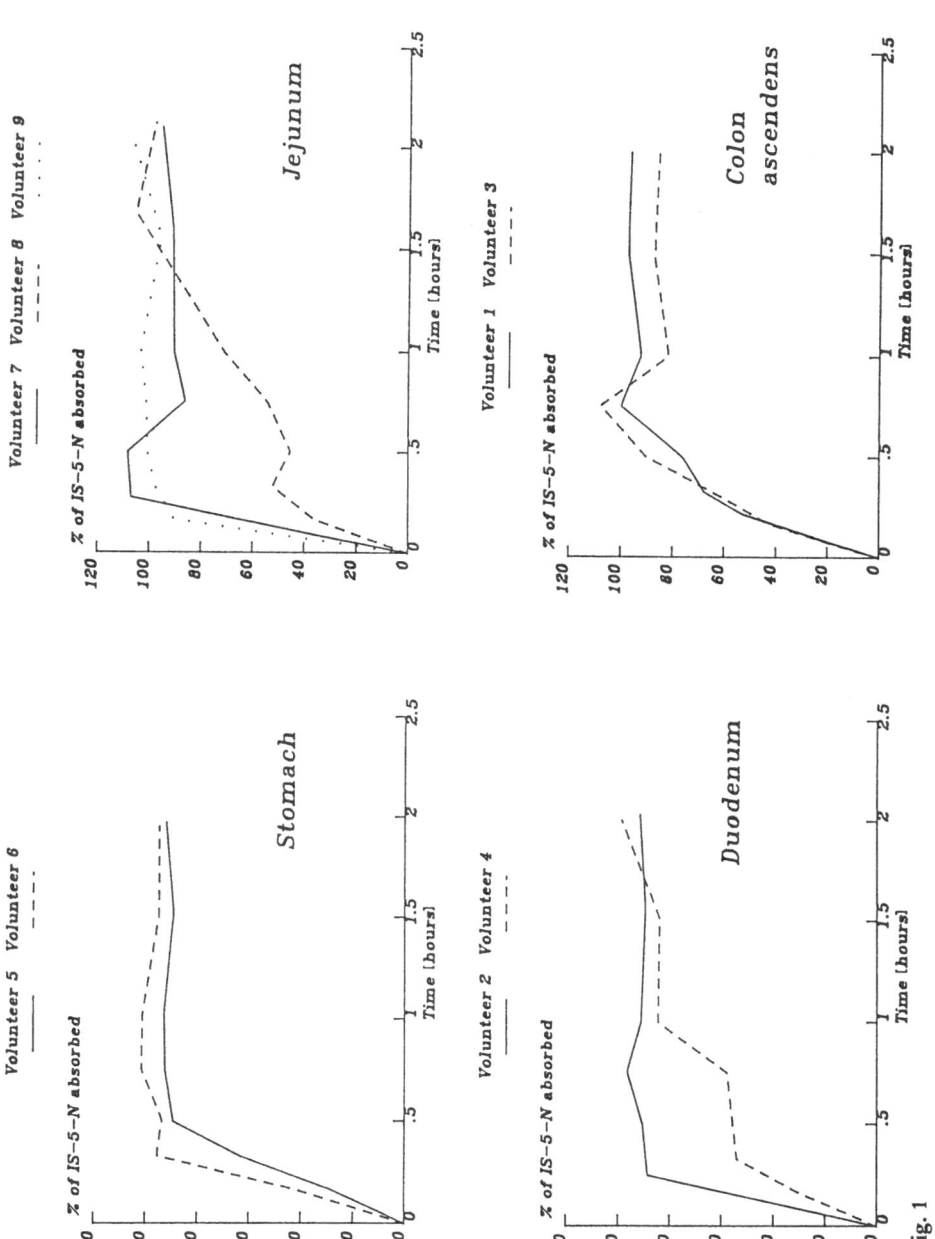

Fig. 1

Absorption of IS-5-N in healthy volunteers after release of the drug from the HF-capsule in different regions of the GI-tract (calculated by the method of Wagner and Nelson).

79

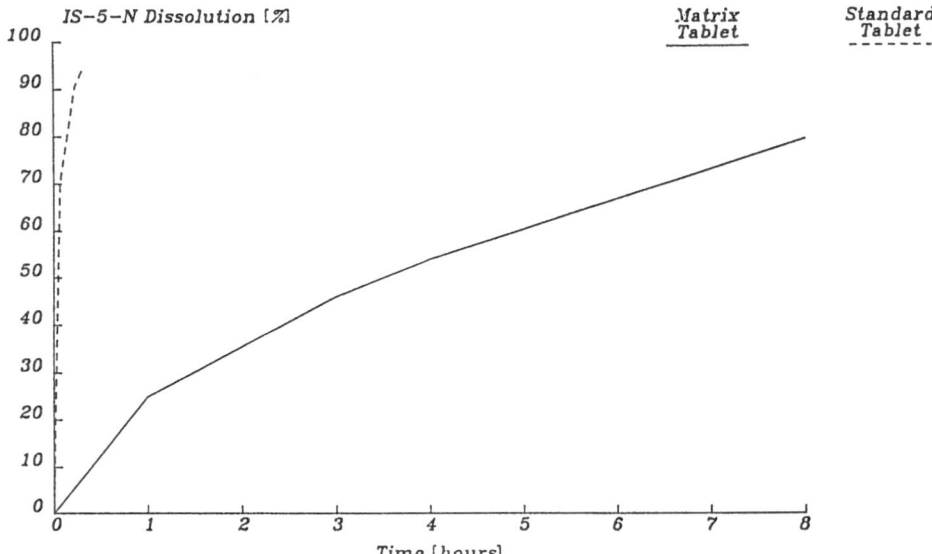

Fig. 2

In vitro release of IS-5-N from a 100 mg matrix tablet and a 40 mg standard tablet (Paddle test according to USPXXI, H$_2$O, 65 RPM).

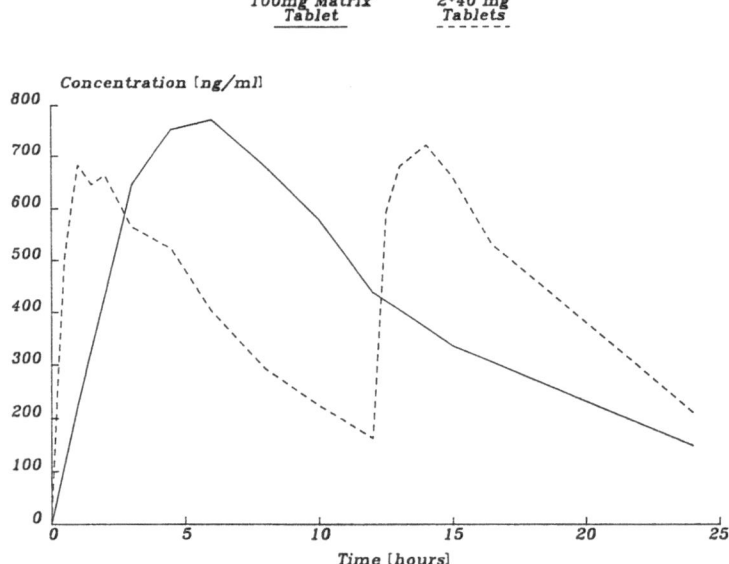

Fig. 3

Mean plasma concentrations of IS-5-N after oral administration of a 100 mg matrix tablet and 2 × 40 mg standard tablets to nine healthy volunteers in an open crossover trial. The doses were ingested following a light standard breakfast.

The final IS-5-N sustained release formulation is a matrix tablet with an in vitro release (Figure 2) characterized by a comparatively rapid phase during the first hour followed by a slower, almost linear phase during the next 4 hours. After 8 hours about 80% of the drug is liberated. A comparative bioavailability study of the new formulation versus 2 × 40 mg standard tablets was performed in healthy volunteers. The mean IS-5-N plasma concentrations are shown in Figure 3. The results confirmed that the objective of a plasma profile being retarded sufficiently to enable once a day treatment was reached, and that the loss of bioavailability could be limited to 20%.

References

[1] F.N. Christensen, S.S. Davis, J.G. Hardy, M.J. Taylor, D.R. Whalley, C.G. Wilson: *J. Pharm. Pharmacol.* **37**, 91−95 (1985).

[2] C.G. Wilson and J.G. Hardy: *J. Pharm. Pharmacol.* **37**, 573−575 (1985).

[3] E.K. Prokop, V.J. Caride, A.R. Marano and R. McCallum: *J. Nucl. Med.* **25**, 97 (1984).

[4] S.S. Davis, J.G. Hardy, M.J. Taylor, D.R. Whalley, C.G. Wilson, *Int. J. Pharmaceutics* **21**, 331−340 (1984).

[5] S.S. Davis, J.G. Hardy, C.G. Wilson, L.C. Feely and K.J. Palin: *Int. J. Pharmaceutics* **32**, 85−90 (1986).

Diskussion

Frage
Welche Ursachen kommen für die verminderte Absorption in der 2. Hälfte des Untersuchungszeitraums in Frage?

Antwort
Die verminderte Absorption wird jenseits der 10. Stunde nach Applikation offenbar durch eine dann erfolgende bakterielle Zersetzung im Darm erklärbar. Eine andere Möglichkeit wäre allerdings, daß tatsächlich die Absorption durch die Wand des Colons reduziert ist. Eine dritte Möglichkeit wäre die Verteilung der Substanz im Darminhalt und deshalb die schlechtere Bereitstellung zur Absorption.

Gastrointestinal Absorption of Drugs: Physico-Chemical and Biomathematical Aspects

D. Brockmeier, H.-G. Grigoleit

Klinische Forschung, Abt. Biometrie
Hoechst AG, D-6230 Frankfurt/Main 80

Abstract

Drug absorption after oral administration — the most convenient and popular way of applying a drug — takes place in both the stomach and the small intestine. Little is known about the absorption characteristics of the colon.

The absorption kinetics of piretanide were investigated in a series of studies. The drug was placed in different parts of the gastrointestinal tract using endoscopic techniques. Preparations for gastroscopy, duodenoscopy and coloscopy followed standard gastroenterological procedures.

The aim of the studies was to determine the rate and extent to which piretanide is absorbed at the different sites of the gastrointestinal tract. The area under the concentration-time data was evaluated as a relative measure of the total amount absorbed following administration at the different sites. The rate of absorption is judged by the total mean time, as the sum of the mean time of absorption and the mean time in the steady-state volume of distribution. Differences in the amount absorbed will be reflected in the area under the curve, and differences in the rate of absorption will be reflected in the total mean time, providing that total clearance from and mean time in the steady-state volume of distribution remain reasonably constant, a property which is clearly met by piretanide.

Based on the pK values and the pH-dependent O/W-partition of piretanide, it is expected that absorption from the stomach is promoted. In contrast, it can be seen from the concentration-time profiles and the pharmacokinetic characteristics evaluated that piretanide is absorbed faster from the duodenum than from the stomach. Hence, the mean time in the duodenum is lower than that for stomach [1]. No differences between the area under the curve were detected for these two sites of administration.

The absorption rate, and probably also the amount absorbed, are markedly lower after placement in the colon [1].

Since it is not clear whether the plasma concentration after instilling piretanide into the stomach arose from drug transported to the duodenum, whence it is absorbed, or from absorption directly from the stomach, piretanide was instilled into the stomach with simultaneous immobilization of the stomach using hyoscine-N-butylbromide. Pronounced interindividual differences were seen in this study indicating that in some subjects piretanide is absorbed directly from the stomach while absorption from the stomach is negligible in others [2].

pH-dependent solubility appears to be the major determinant of absorption for piretanide. The solubility of the drug is lowest in the stomach, where under fasting conditions the pH may be between 2 and 3. The rate and/or onset of absorption from this site obviously reflects this. A further important factor is gastric motility, and thus gastric emptying. When gastric motility is inhibited by hyoscine-N-butylbromide, the absorption is clearly biphasic, reflecting the pH-dependent solubility and gastric emptying time [2].

In summary, studying physico-chemical properties of individual substances provides valuable information for the design of a formulation, and in particular sustained release formulations. However, absorption of the drug from different sites along the gastrointestinal tract must be determined, in order to tailor the formulation to the required release pattern. Although all parts of the gastrointestinal tract may be capable of absorbing the agent, significant differences between the rates of absorption may exist. Thus, total contact time may become a decisive variable for drug availability.

References

[1] D. Brockmeier, H.-G. Grigoleit, H. Leonhardt: The absorption of piretanide from the gastrointestinal tract is site-dependent. *Eur. J. Clin. Pharmacol.* **30**, 79–82 (1986).
[2] D. Brockmeier, H.-G. Grigoleit, H. Heptner, B.H. Meyer: Kinetics of piretanide absorption from the gastrointestinal tract. *Meth. and Find. Exptl. Pharmacol.* **8** (12), 731–739 (1986).

Diskussion

Frage
Nach Untersuchungen der Arbeitsgruppe um Winne ist die Gültigkeit der Verteilungshypothese eher die Ausnahme denn die Regel. Trifft dies für die vorgetragenen Ergebnisse zu?

Antwort
Die Verteilungshypothese beschreibt nicht ausreichend die real bei der Absorption vorliegenden Bedingungen, da sie nur für Gleichgewichtsbedingungen gilt. Dies ist im Fall der intestinalen Absorption jedoch nie der Fall, da kreislaufseitig die Einstellung eines Gleichgewichts ausgeschlossen werden kann („Sinkbedingungen"). Ferner sind die erforderlichen Zeitkonstanten für Dissoziation und Reassoziation so klein, daß beide Prozesse nicht mehr geschwindigkeitsbestimmend sein können.
In Hinweisen aus dem Auditorium wird festgestellt, daß die mit den klassischen physiko-chemischen Methoden (Oktanol-Wasser-Verteilungskoeffizient) gewonnenen Daten keine ausreichende Grundlage für die mehrfaktoriellen Vorgänge bei der Absorption sein können, da z.B. die Aufnahmekapazität der lipophilen Phase so nicht erfaßt werden kann. Diese in vitro-Daten haben deshalb nur den Charakter von Interpretationshilfen.
In einer weiteren Diskussionsbemerkung wird dagegen gesetzt, daß unter Berücksichtigung mehrerer pKa-Werte und des Verteilungs- und Lösungsverhaltens doch fundierte Aussagen erhalten werden. Diese Frage wird anschließend in Analogie zur Eiweißbindung und zu den Eliminationsvorgängen in der Leber und deren Geschwindigkeitskonstanten unter verschiedenen Bedingungen diskutiert.

Absorption of Hexobarbital und Caffeine in Patients with Liver Cirrhosis

R. Joeres, H. Klinker, G. Hofstetter, W. Zilly, E. Richter

Medizinische Universitätsklinik, Josef-Schneider-Straße 2,
D-8700 Würzburg and Hartwaldklinik der BfA, D-8788 Bad Brückenau

Summary

Hexobarbital and caffeine elimination is impaired in patients with hepatitis and liver cirrhosis according to the severity of the disease. However, absorption of both substances is not altered in patients with liver disease.

Zusammenfassung

Koffein- und Hexobarbitalelimination können als Maß für die Leberfunktionseinschränkung bei Patienten mit Hepatitis und Lebercirrhose herangezogen werden. Die Absorption (k_A) beider Substanzen wird jedoch durch Lebererkrankungen mit und ohne portale Hypertension nicht beeinflußt. Veränderungen von C_{max} und t_{max} sind Folge einer Abnahme der Eliminationsgeschwindigkeit (k_E). Der Ausdruck $AUC \times k_E$ liefert vergleichbare Werte für die Vollständigkeit der Absorption von Koffein und belegt die erhöhte Bioverfügbarkeit von Hexobarbital bei Lebererkrankungen bedingt durch eine Abnahme des first-pass-Effektes.

Introduction

Hexobarbital and caffeine elimination are a measure of the oxidative drug metabolizing capacity in patients with liver disease, since both substrates are almost completely metabolized by the liver [1, 2]. Delayed gastric emptying, however, leads to incomplete absorption [3].

Liver diseases with portal hypertension result in changes of the gastro-intestinal hemodynamics with alterations of the intestinal motility and may possibly induce functional disorders of the intestinal mucosa. Our study was performed in order to obtain data on the absorption of hexobarbital and caffeine in patients with liver cirrhosis and hepatitis in comparison to a control group without liver disease.

Methods

Patients with viral or toxic hepatitis and posthepatitic or alcoholic cirrhosis received 250 mg hexobarbital or 366 mg caffeine orally after an overnight fast. Blood samples were taken before and 15 min, 30 min, 1 h, 2 h, 4 h, 8 h, 12 h and 24 h after application of the drugs. Healthy volunteers provided control data. Measurement of hexobarbital and caffeine plasma levels was performed by gas-chromatography [4, 5]. Calculation of pharmacokinetic parameters was carried out using the PEROS computer programm from ICS Company Information and Communication Systems Marketing GmbH, 6000 Frankfurt/M., FRG, under the assumption of an open one-compartment-model and first order absorption kinetics. The areas under the plasma concentration-time curves were standardized by multiplying AUC by k_E (AUC $\times$ k_E). Arithmetically, AUC $\times$ k_E corresponds to $C_O = D/V_D$ and is a mesure for bioavailability when groups of patients with considerably diverging elimination rates are compared to each other.

Statistical calculations were performed using the Wilcoxon U-test.

Results

The reduction of caffeine elimination in patients with liver disease is accompanied by a decrease of k_E and a corresponding increase in AUC. These changes are more pronounced in liver cirrhosis than in hepatitis (Table 1). The volume of distribution, however, is not changed. The product of AUC $\times$ k_E also remains unchanged. K_A shows no disease dependent changes, and in the three groups C_{max} increases only slightly with the reduction in the elimination rate. In contrast, t_{max} of caffeine in liver cirrhosis is considerably delayed when compared to the control group, whereas in patients with hepatitis intermediate values are found.

With hexobarbital, elimination also decreases according to the severity of the liver disease. AUC increases correspondingly. The product of AUC $\times$ k_E, however, in contrast to caffeine, is increased in patients with liver disease when compared to the control group. On the other hand, the apparent volume of distribution is reduced in these patients (Table 2). The absorption rate constant k_A and t_{max} show no disease dependent changes. C_{max} is increased in patients with liver disease according to the severity of the disease.

Table 1. Pharmacokinetic parameters of orally administered caffeine (366 mg) in the control group, in patients with hepatitis and in patients with cirrhosis of the liver

	C_{max} (µg/ml)	t_{max} (min)	k_A (min^{-1})	k_E (min^{-1})	AUC (µg $\times$ min $\times$ ml^{-1})	AUC $\times$ k_E (µg/ml)	V_D (l)
control group	9.43	77	0.0762	0.0025	5361	11.34	35
n = 13	± 2.44	± 50	±0.0660	±0.0011	± 2889	± 3.05	±11
hepatitis	10.12	95	0.0564	0.0022	8486	11.45	33
n = 14	± 3.21	± 78	±0.0533	±0.0016	± 6258	± 1.83	± 5
liver cirrhosis	10.90	125*	0.0625	0.0007***	49005***	11.77	35
n = 14	± 4.26	± 93	±0.0452	±0.0005	±74503	± 4.58	±12

mean values ± SD; * p <0.05 vs control group; *** vs hepatitis

Table 2. Pharmacokinetic parameters of orally administered hexobarbital (250 mg) in the control group, in patients with hepatitis and in patients with cirrhosis of the liver

	C_{max} (μg/ml)	t_{max} (min)	k_A (min^{-1})	k_E (min^{-1})	AUC (μg $\times$ min $\times$ ml^{-1})	AUC $\times$ k_E (μg/ml)	V_D (l)
control group n = 10	0.98 ±0.38	195 ± 60	0.0226 ±0.0187	0.0037 ±0.0028	597 ± 377	1.57 ±0.73	197 ± 72
hepatitis n = 18	1.74* ±0.61	141 ± 66	0.0329 ±0.0252	0.0016* ±0.0006	1794* ±2042	2.24* ±0.89	133* ± 55
liver cirrhosis n = 24	2.22*** ±0.61	152 ± 83	0.0425 ±0.0494	0.0011*** ±0.0005	2951*** ±1420	2.69*** ±0.87	107* ± 38

mean values ± SD; * p <0.05 vs control group; ** vs hepatitis

Discussion

A decrease in hexobarbital and caffeine elimination in patients with liver disease could be demonstrated. The parameters describing the rate and completeness of absorption can be interpreted easier in the case of caffeine, which is a low-clearance substance, than for hexobarbital. Because of the differing elimination rates, the AUCs do not provide suitable data for evaluating completeness of absorption. Only the product of AUC $\times$ k_E, which corresponds arithmetically to $C_0 = D/V_D$, indicates that caffeine is completely absorbed in all three groups [6]. Our results show no differences in the rate of absorption k_A. The slight increase in C_{max} and the significant delay in t_{max} are sufficiently explained by the Bateman function as a consequence of the decrease in k_E and provide no evidence of an impairment of absorption.

For hexobarbital, however, interpretation of pharmacokinetic parameters is more difficult because of the relatively high clearance (in healthy volunteers 620 ± 429 ml/min) in comparison with the liver blood flow (about 1000−1500 ml/min) and the extensive presystemic elimination because of the first pass effect. Thus the decrease in the apparent volume of distribution accompanied by the decrease in the clearance and corresponding increase in AUC $\times$ k_E is a consequence of an increase in bioavailibility due to reduced presystemic elimination. This also explains the considerably higher peak plasma concentrations (C_{max}) in patients with liver disease compared to healthy volunteers. In contrast, absorption rate k_A and t_{max} are not affected and thus reflecting an unchanged absorption in liver disease with and without portal hypertension.

Changes in pharmacokinetic parameters of caffeine and hexobarbital in patients with liver disease can be interpreted as a consequence of reduced elimination without any indication that absorption is altered.

With the support of the Deutsche Forschungsgemeinschaft.

References

[1] E. Renner, H. Wietholtz, P. Huguenin, M.J. Arnaud, R. Preisig: Caffeine: A model compound for Measuring liver function. *Hepatology* **4**, 38–46 (1984).

[2] D.D. Breimer, W. Zilly, E. Richter: Pharmacokinetics of hexobarbital in acute hepatitis and after apparent recovery. *Clin. Pharmacol. Ther.* **18**, 433–440 (1975).

[3] D. Brachtel, E. Richter: Coffein-Resorption bei Patienten mit Magenentleerungsstörungen. Siehe diesen Band Seite 108.

[4] D.D. Breimer, J.M. van Rossum: Rapid and sensitive gaschromatographic determination of hexobarbital in plasma of man using a nitrogen detector. *J. Chromatography* **88**, 235–243 (1974).

[5] H. Heusler, E. Richter: Quantitative Bestimmung von Coffein in biologischen Flüssigkeiten mit Hilfe der Gaschromatographie und N-selektiver Detektion in N. Rietbrock, B.G. Woodcook, A.H. Staib, *Theophylline and other Methylxanthines*, Vieweg & Sohn, Braunschweig (1982).

[6] J. Blanchard, S.J.A. Sawers: The absolute bioavailibility of caffeine in man. *Eur. J. Clinical Pharmacol.* **24**, 93–98 (1983).

Influence of Absorption Rate on the Metabolic Kinetics of Theophylline

S.A. Hotchkiss, J. Caldwell,
Department of Pharmacology, St. Mary's Hospital Medical School,
London W2 1PG, U.K.

Summary

Theophylline is administered orally to patients primarily in the form of sustained-release preparations. In view of the widespread use of these formulations and the non-linear kinetics reported to exist for theophylline, it is important to assess the effect of slow delivery upon the metabolic kinetics of the drug. If certain metabolic pathways are saturated when a conventional preparation is administered, this may occur as a result of the immediate high concentration of drug reaching the liver overwhelming the enzymes responsible for metabolism. If this is the case, one might expect that if a drug is delivered slowly to the liver, as occurs when a sustained-release preparation is administered, this may not saturate the metabolic pathway concerned and hence metabolism will not become zero-order.

Single doses of conventional and sustained-release theophylline preparations were administered to 5 healthy volunteers on separate occasions. After conventional preparations, high plasma theophylline levels were observed, together with zero-order elimination of the 3 major metabolites, 3-methylxanthine, 1-methyluric acid and 1,3-dimethyluric acid. Plasma levels were lower after roughly equivalent doses of sustained-release theophylline, and elimination was only observed to become zero-order for the metabolite 3-methylxanthine.

These observations indicate that the rate of absorption of theophylline from the gastrointestinal tract can affect its pharmacokinetic disposition. This may be of significance in the clinical situation for the safe and effective use of theophylline in the management of asthma.

Introduction

Enzymic metabolism is an important determinant of the pharmacokinetic profile of many drugs. Enzyme kinetics follow the Michaelis-Menten equation, with the rate of conversion of metabolite(s) being a function of enzyme affinity and concentration and the concentration of drug, such that the rate becomes constant above certain substrate concentrations.

There have been a number of reports that the pharmacokinetics of theophylline are dose-dependent, arising from observations of a disproportionate increase in plasma concentration with increasing dose (non-linear kinetics) [1, 2]. More specifically, certain authors have found that the plasma elimination kinetics for theophylline are dose-dependent within the therapeutic dose range [3], which has been explained in terms of the saturation of metabolic pathways.

Monks et al. [4, 5] reported that the rate and extent of theophylline metabolism was enhanced when other methylxanthines were removed from the diet, possibly due to saturation of the N-demethylation pathway giving rise to 3-methylxanthine by the normal body pool (ca. 300 mg) of methylxanthines. Other authors have presented evidence for the occurrence of non-linear elimination kinetics for all three major theophylline metabolites [3, 6].

Considering the fact that there are a great variety of sustained-release preparations of theophylline in widespread use, it is surprising that the influence of delivery rate upon the kinetics of its metabolism has not been investigated. It is possible that delayed, slowed or prolonged absorption may affect the metabolic disposition of certain drugs, especially where saturation of metabolic pathways or first-pass metabolism are involved.

When a conventional theophylline preparation is adminstered, from which absorption is rapid and complete, high concentrations of the drug will reach the liver which may saturate the enzymes responsible for metabolism. However, if absorption is retarded, and the drug is delivered more slowly to the liver, as occurs when a sustained-release preparation is administered, saturation of these metabolic pathway(s) may not occur and metabolism will not become zero-order.

The present study was designed to investigate the effect of absorption rate upon the metabolic kinetics of theophylline in healthy human volunteers. In order to achieve different rates of absorption, both conventional and sustained-release formulations of theophylline were administered, the former giving immediate and the latter delayed delivery to the site of metabolism.

Materials and Methods

Conventional-release aminophylline (theophylline ethylenediamine) tablets (100 mg Aminophylline BP containing 80 mg theophylline) and controlled-release aminophylline (350 mg Phyllocontin Forte containing 280 mg theophylline) were used in the study. 5 healthy volunteers (3M, 2F, 23–37 y; 54–70 kg) received each medication orally on separate occasions after an overnight fast and 4 days abstention from all dietary methylxanthines. Food was withheld for 2 hours after dosing. Serial blood and urine samples were taken up to 30 h and theophylline in plasma was determined by the HPLC method of Cotgreave & Caldwell [7], and theophylline and metabolites in urine were determined by the HPLC method of Hotchkiss & Caldwell [8].

Results

Maximum plasma levels (C_{max}) of theophylline were achieved after 1.5–3 h with the conventional tablets, and were up to 3 times greater than after the sustained-release preparation (eg. 11.1 vs. 3.4 µg/ml), the latter being achieved only after 10 h. When C_{max} values were corrected for dose they were significantly lower (by 100%) after the sustained release formulation.

From plasma concentration-time graphs (Fig. 1) the elimination phase of theophylline was monoexponential. Although the elimination rate constant (k) appeared to be smaller

Concentration ($\mu g\ ml^{-1}$)

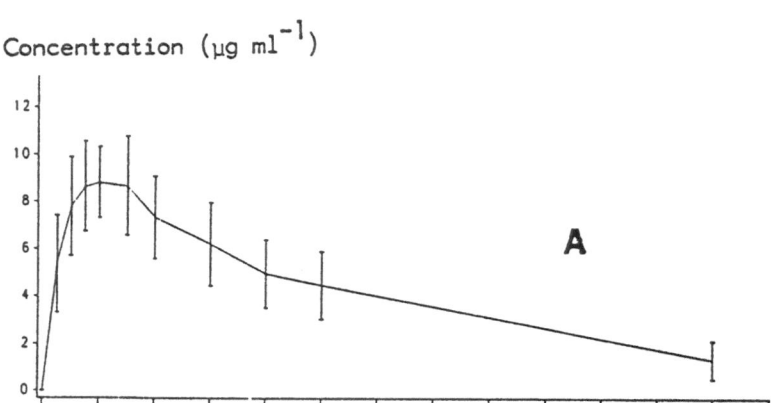

Time (h)

Concentration ($\mu g\ ml^{-1}$)

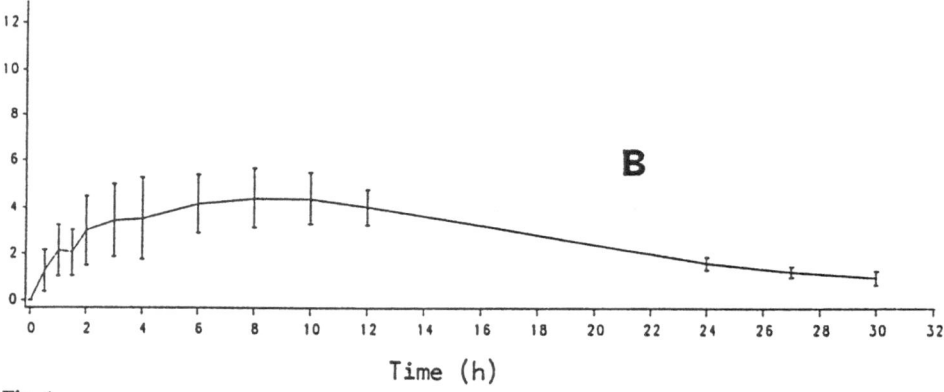

Time (h)

Fig. 1

Mean ($\pm$ SD; n = 5) plasma concentration – time curves after administration of (a) conventional theophylline and (B) sustained-release theophylline.

with the sustained-release tablets, there were no statistically significant differences in k and $t_{1/2}$ between the preparations (Table 1).

AUC_{24} and AUC_{∞} when corrected for dose were not significantly different between the formulations. There were no significant differences between preparations for renal, metabolic or total theophylline clearance or volume of distribution (Table 1).

The 0–48 h urinary recovery of theophylline was 83% and 80% after conventional and sustained-release theophylline respectively. The pattern of urinary metabolites was not influenced by the rate of delivery (Table 2).

90

Table 1. Pharmacokinetic parameters determined for both conventional and sustained-release theophylline. (Mean ± S.D., n = 5)

		Conventional Theophylline	Sustained-release Theophylline
k	(h^{-1})	0.091 ± 0.019	0.073 ± 0.013
$t_{1/2}$	(h)	8.0 ± 2.0	9.8 ± 1.8
* C_{max}	(µg/ml)	30.3 ± 4.7	16.1 ± 4.3
t_{max}	(h)	1.9 ± 0.7	7.4 ± 3.0
* AUC_{24}	(µg h/ml)	329.4 ± 93.4	277.1 ± 69.6
* $AUC\infty$	(µg h/ml)	383.4 ± 136.9	356.4 ± 71.8
CL_T	(ml/h/kg)	44.8 ± 14.9	44.6 ± 4.4
CL_r	(ml/h/kg)	5.2 ± 3.5	4.7 ± 1.4
CL_m	(ml/h/kg)	39.6 ± 12.6	39.9 ± 5.3
V_D	(L/kg)	0.49 ± 0.07	0.62 ± 0.11
* Values expressed per g theophylline			

Table 2. 0−48 h urinary excretion (% dose) of theophylline and metabolites after conventional and sustained-release preparations. (Mean ± S.D., n= 5)

	Conventional Theophylline	Sustained-release Theophylline
1-Methyluric acid	17.3 ± 4.8	17.3 ± 3.5
3-Methylxanthine	11.1 ± 2.8	10.6 ± 3.2
1,3-Dimethyluric acid	43.7 ± 1.0	41.2 ± 5.7
Theophylline	11.4 ± 5.3	10.8 ± 3.8
Total	83.5 ± 3.9	79.9 ± 9.3

After conventional tablets, log excretion rate-time graphs for all metabolites exhibited plateaus, indicating a constant excretion rate, for up to 12 h after administration, i.e. zero-order elimination. However, urinary theophylline excretion followed first-order kinetics. After the sustained-release tablets, the rate of excretion of metabolites increased as absorption continued for up to 5 h, reaching a plateau which was maintained for up 12−24 h, and therefore declined in a log-linear fashion.

From the Hanes analysis [4], it appeared that the conversions to 3-methylxanthine, 1-methyluric acid and 1,3-dimethyluric acid were all saturated after the conventional preparation. However, only the formation of 3-methylxanthine appeared to be saturated after the sustained-release preparation.

When theophylline was given in conventional tablets the rate of urinary excretion of metabolites increased with increasing theophylline plasma concentration to maximum rates, which occurred at 7 µg/ml theophylline for both 1-methyluric acid and 1,3-dimethyluric acid, but was less than 4 µg/ml for 3-methylxanthine. After sustained-release theophylline, as before its conversion to 3-methylxanthine was saturated at plasma levels of less than 4 µg/ml theophylline. However, the excretion rates of the other compounds did not reach a maximum, but increased linearly with increasing theophylline plasma concentration. These observations are accounted for by the fact that theophylline plasma levels did not rise above the level (7 µg/ml) necessary for the saturation of the processes for the urinary excretion of 1,3-dimethyl- and 1-methyl-uric acids.

Discussion

Comparison of both the plasma elimination kinetics of theophylline, and the quantities of the drug and its metabolites recovered in the 0—48 h urine, after both conventional and sustained-release theophylline tablets suggest that the rate of delivery of this drug has no meaningful effect upon its disposition.

However, from a more detailed consideration of the rates of metabolite elimination and their relationships with the plasma concentrations of theophylline, it can be seen that the rate of elimination of 3-methylxanthine, 1,3-dimethyluric acid and 1-methyluric acid are described by Michaelis-Menten kinetics, being saturable at therapeutic plasma concentrations of theophylline. Only the most readily saturable pathway, the 1-N-demethylation of 3-methylxanthine, was saturated when the sustained-release preparation was given, since plasma theophylline levels did not reach the concentration (7 µg/ml) necessary to saturate the process(es) leading to the elimination of 1-methyluric acid and 1,3-dimethyl-uric acid. However, the concentration necessary to saturate the conversion to 3-methylxanthine (~ 4 µg/ml) was readily achieved.

Acknowledgements

This work was supported by a grant from Napp Laboratories Ltd. We thank Professor R.L. Smith for this continued encouragement of work in this area.

References

[1] R.J. Ogilvie: Clinical pharmacokinetics of theophylline. *Clin. Pharmacokinet.*, **3**, 267—293 (1978).
[2] L. Hendeles, M. Weinberger, G. Johnson: Monitoring serum theophylline levels. *Clin. Pharmacokinet.*, **3**, 294—312 (1978).
[3] J.H.G. Jonkman, D.D.S. Tang-Lui, R.A. Upton, S. Riegelman: Measurement of the excretion characteristics of theophylline and its major metabolites. *Eur. J. Clin. Pharmacol.*, **20**, 435—441 (1981).
[4] T.J. Monks, J. Caldwell, R.L. Smith: Influence of methylxanthine-containing foods on theophylline metabolism and kinetics. *Clin. Pharmacol. Ther.*, **26**, 513—524 (1979).
[5] T.J. Monks, C.A. Lawrie, J. Caldwell: The effect of increased caffeine intake on the metabolism and pharmacokinetics of theophylline in man. *Biopharm. Drug Disp.*, **2**, 31—37 (1981).
[6] D.D.S. Lui Tang, R.L. Williams, S. Riegelman: Non-linear theophylline elimination. *Clin. Pharmacol. Ther.*, **31**, 358—369 (1982).
[7] I.A. Cotgreave, J. Caldwell: Comparative plasma pharmacokinetics of theophylline & ethylenediamine after the administration of aminophylline to man. *J. Pharm. Pharmacol.*, **35**, 378—382 (1983).
[8] S.A. Hotchkiss, J. Caldwell: A high pressure liquid chromatographic assay for theophylline and its major metabolites in human urine. *J. Chromatog.* (1987) In press.

Metabolism of Fosfestrol by Intestinal Mucosa

H. Oelschläger, D. Rothley

Institut für Pharmaz. Chemie, Johann Wolfgang Goethe-Universität, D-6000 Frankfurt

Summary

The formation of E-DES-monoglucuronide by the liver enzymes may be almost completely hindered by oral administration of a substance x, which does not influence the conjugation capacity of the intestinal mucosa. The structure of x is known but will be published later.

Fosfestrol (Honvan[R])[1] is mainly metabolised by cleaving its two phosphate ester groups in the intestinal mucosa by hydrolysis; the diethylstilbestrol formed is then conjugated (glucuronide and sulphate). After almost completely, but reversibly blocking the conjugating capacity of the liver by administering a substance x, evidence by analysis of the plasma metabolites was obtained after intravenous and oral administration. The amount of conjugates found in human plasma after intravenous application was negligible, but substantial quantities were seen after oral application (Fig. 1).

Measurements of fosfestrol and its metabolites were possible due to the development of a specific sample preparation procedure and a new measuring technique. After simultaneous addition of tetrabutyl-ammonium phosphate and methanol with subsequent precipi-

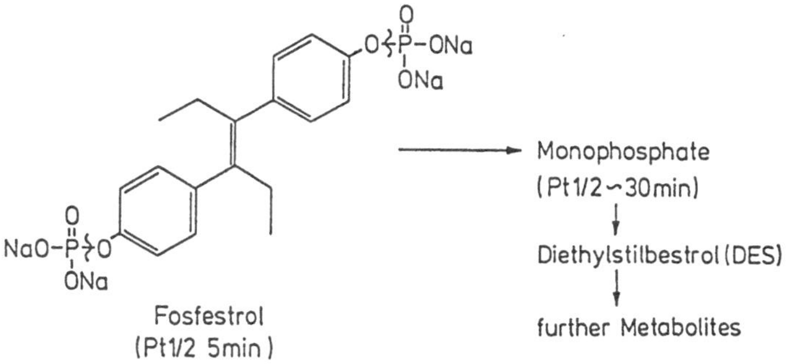

Fig. 1
Enzymatic cleavage of fosfestrol.

---

1 Manufacturer: Degussa Pharma-Gruppe Asta-Werke AG, Bielefeld, FRG.

tation of plasma proteins and formation of ion pairs the metabolites were extracted from plasma with recovery rates >90%. Depending on the structure quantitative determination was carried out by either UV-measurement at 236 nm or by the use of an electrochemical detector at + 1V (acetonitrile/phosphate buffer (pH 3.1) 1:1). The main feature of the 3-electrodes measuring cell is a carbon paste electrode that we have developed ourselves and which work for at least 12 months trouble-free without needing to clean it.

For experimental details and results compare:

References

H. Oelschläger: Krebschemotherapeutika aus pharmakokinetischer Sicht. In: *Schriftenreihe der Bundesapothekerkammer zur wissenschaftlichen Fortbildung*, Bd. XII/Gelbe Reihe, 41 (1984).

H. Oelschläger: Fosfestrol: Pharmakokinetische Untersuchungen. In: *Pharmazeutische Zeitung*, **129**, 2271 (1984).

H. Oelschläger, et al.: Plasmaspiegel von Fosfestrol und seinem Monophosphat, von Diethylstilbestrol und seinem Monoglucuronid nach intravenöser Gabe bei Patienten mit metastasierendem Prostatakarzinom. In: *Arzneimittel-Forschung/Drug Research*, **34**, 1333 (1984).

H. Oelschläger, et al.: Direkte Bestimmung von Diethylstilbestrol und seinen Monokonjugaten im Plasma. In: *Arzneimittel-Forschung/Drug Research*, **36**, 759 (1986).

H. Oelschläger, et al.: Plasmakonzentrationen von Fosfestrol sowie von Diethylstilbestrol und seinen Konjugaten nach intravenöser Gabe an Prostatakarzinom-Patienten. In: *Arzneimittel-Forschung/Drug Research*, **36**, 1284 (1986).

D. Rothley, H. Oelschläger: Direkte Approximation von Plasma-Konzentrations-Zeit-Kurven des E-Diethylstilbestrol-Monoglucuronids nach oraler und i.v. Gabe von Fosfestrol. In: *Pharmazie*, **41**, 862 (1986).

Drug Input Rate from the GI-Tract.
Michaelis-Menten Kinetics and the Bioavailability
of Slow-Release Verapamil and Nifedipine

B.G. Woodcock, G. Menke, A. Fischer, H. Köhne[1], N. Rietbrock
Department of Clinical Pharmacology, University Clinic Frankfurt, Theodor-Stern-Kai 7,
D-6000 Frankfurt am Main
[1]Dr. Rentschler, Arzneimittel GmbH & Co., Mittelstrasse 18, D-7958 Laupheim

Summary

1. This paper presents evidence from studies with slow release verapamil and nifedipine for Michaelis-Menten metabolism during first pass through the liver. Drug input rate from the GI-tract after an oral dose appears to be a determinant of biovailability. Highest oral bioavailabilities are observed with standard release formulations at high dosage. The bioavailability of slow release formulations with a zero order release kinetic is lower than standard release formulations and related to the dissolution rate in vitro.

2. The presence of non-linear absorption kinetics offers a further explanation for the considerable inter-patient variability in AUC since the ability of drug to cross the liver is a function of the concentrations attained in portal blood which will be dependent on dissolution conditions prevailing in the GI-tract.

3. Depending on the choice of the dose and dosage interval of the conventional release formulation used for comparison, and as a consequence of Michaelis-Menten first pass metabolism, it is possible to obtain relative bioavailability data showing superiority, equivalence, or biovailability loss with the slow release form. This may explain the discrepancies in bioavailability data for slow release drugs reported in the literature.

4. 'True' estimates of relative bioavailability of a slow release formulation can only be achieved if:
   a) Steady state conditions are present.
   b) The dose and dosage interval of the slow and conventional release formulation are the same.

5. Since a slower dissolution rate is 'ipso facto' associated with a lower bioavailability, slow release formulations of verapamil and nifedipine cannot be classified as being 'inferior' or of poorer quality on the basis of bioavailability alone.

Introduction

The bioavailability of many slow release drugs used in cardiovascular therapy is lower than that for the standard (conventional) release formulations. This has been observed in the case of β-blockers, calcium antagonists and long acting nitrates. There are several possible explanations for this phenomenon e.g. increased bacterial metabolism and poor absorption in the lower bowel, but there is little or no evidence to show that these explanations are valid. Metoprolol, a lipophilic drugs with marked first pass metabolism is well absorbed in the colon despite the relatively low surface area of the lumen and the high microflora concentrations in this section of the GI-tract (Hirtz, this volume). The rectal absorption of propranolol is greater than after oral application [1]. On the other hand Koch-Weser and Schechter [2] have stated that for drugs undergoing first pass metabolism: 'The percentage of the dose that reaches the systemic circulation unchanged may decrease as the rate of intestinal absorption is slowed. In extreme cases a drug can thus almost totally lose its bioavailability by the oral route'.

The theoretical basis for non-linear first pass metabolism was subsequently reported by Wagner [3], who showed that the first pass metabolism of orally administered propranolol is dependent on the rate of drug input. The equations derived were based on Michaelis-Menten kinetics and involved calculation of V_{max} and K_{max}. The equations predicted the findings of Dvornick et al. [4] who observed that the bioavailability at steady state of conventional release propranolol tablets given as 40 mg twice daily was 30% higher than when the same dose was applied as 20 mg doses 4 times daily. They also explained the observations of Garg et al. [5] and Ohashi et al. [6] who obtained bioavailability values for slow release propranolol formulations of 55% and 51% when compared with the same daily dose of conventional tablets. Wagner [7] has expressed the view that 'essentially all drugs that exert a significant first pass effect will exhibit such non-linear Michaelis-Menten kinetics after oral administration at dose rates in the therapeutic range, as a result of the high drug concentrations entering the liver with this route compared with those after intravenous administration'.

This paper presents evidence, from pharmacokinetic studies on slow release formulations, for Michaelis-Menten first pass metabolism of the calcium antagonists verapamil and nifedipine. The significance of these findings for bioavailability studies is discussed.

Drug Absorption into Portal/Splanchnic Blood: Effect of Delivery Rate and the Concept of an "Oral Bolus Dose"

Passage of lipiphilic cardiovascular drugs across the intestinal wall is thought to be a passive first order process. For drugs which are well absorbed e.g. paracetamol and verapamil (absorption quotient close to 100%; Shomerus et al. [8]) the halftime of absorption of a solution from the GI-tract into portal blood is estimated to be about 7 minutes [9]. Thus the rate of appearance of drug in portal and splanchnic blood and the rate of delivery of drug to the hepatic sinusoids is dependent on the concentration of dissolved drug in the intestinal lumen. For solid oral forms the appearance of drug in blood is slower than this because of the need for dissolution. The absorption halftime with capsules is 0.27 h [10] and with oral dragees 0.95 h [11]. When the dissolution rate is relatively high, as in tablets or capsules with conventional release characteristics, the contents are released rapidly, 80—100% within 30 minutes, a process referred to by Wagner [3] as 'oral bolus

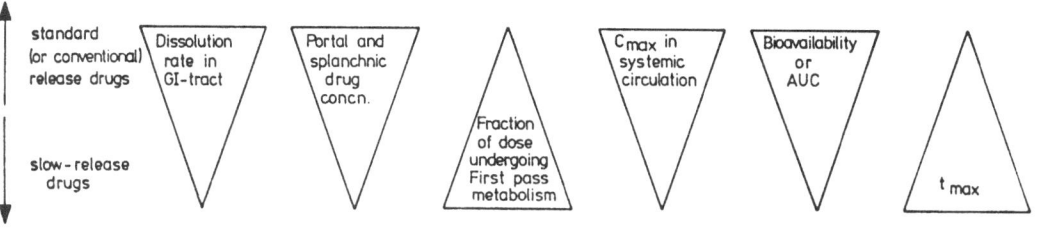

Fig. 1

Pharmacokinetic attributes of slow and conventional release formulations of first pass drugs.

drug delivery', and portal blood levels are high. If first pass metabolism obeys Michaelis-Menten kinetics then progressively increasing the 'bolus dose' should result in an increase in AUC per mg dose administered. When the dissolution rate is slow with a zero order kinetic as in slow release formulations the concentration of dissolved drug in the intestinal lumen is low and relatively constant. As a consequence concentrations in portal blood will be low, first pass extraction high, resulting in a low bioavailability. These pharmacokinetic attributes of slow and conventional release formulations are shown diagramatically in Fig. 1. Some formulations show mixed released characteristics in which part e.g. 30%, of the tablet or capsule contents are released rapidly as a 'bolus' dose. Such formulations would be expected to show intermediate characteristics.

Theoretical Basis for Michaelis-Menten First Pass Kinetics Using the Example of Propranolol

The theoretical basis for describing Michaelis-Menten behaviour of first pass drugs has been reported by Wagner [3, 7] and the symbols used in these reports have been retained in the following brief synopsis. The equations derived appear suitable for calculation of C_{ss} and therefore AUC during zero order input with slow release formulations and also when drug input is irregular and not zero order as in the case of spaced doses of conventional formulations.

1. Saturation of First Pass Metabolism with Increase in Dose

The presence of Michaelis-Menten behaviour of a first pass drug is apparent from the curvilinear relationship between the steady state bioavailability (F_{ss}) and the drug input rate to the body (R_0) (Fig. 2) calculated using:

$$F_{ss} = \frac{1}{1 + \dfrac{V_m - R_0}{Q_L K_m}} \qquad (1)$$

where V_m = maximal velocity of metabolism
K_m = Michaelis-Menten constant
Q_L = Liver blood flow (Assumed to be 1.5 L/min)

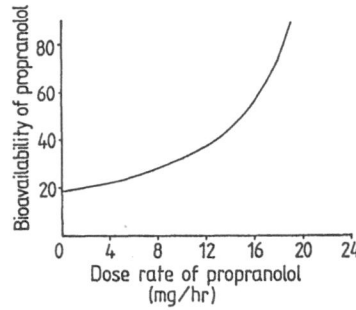

Fig. 2
Plot of propranolol bioavailability against the zero order drug input rate determined using estimated values for K_m and V_m by Wagner [3].

This equation indicates that the intrinsic bioavailability of propranolol (i.e. the biovaliability extrapolated to a zero order input rate of zero) is predicted to be about 20%. Bioavailability increases as R_0 increases until bioavailability approaches 100%. When R_0 is equal to V_m, namely approximately 20 mg/h or 500 mg/day, $F_{ss} = 1$. The calculated bioavailability (25−35%) for bolus doses of 80 mg given three times daily, representing an input rate approaching 10 mg/h, were comparable to the experimentally observed range of values (18−45%) found in six subjects [3].

V_m and K_m required for calculation of this curve were determined from steady state data by obtaining a fit to eq. (2) using experimentally determined values for C_{ss} and R_0 and the method of Wilkinson [12]:

$$C_{ss} = \frac{K_m\,R_0}{V_m - R_0} \tag{2}$$

The equation is applicable to both one- and two-compartment models when there is zero-order input by mouth and can also be applied when input is irregular and not zero-order. Since the intrinsic clearance Cl_i is given by V_m/K_m, V_m and K_m for propranolol could also be derived from single dose clearance data after a low doses of propranolol and the steady state clearance, (Cl_{ss}) [7]; see also eq. (6) Appendix).

2. Zero Order Input and Relative Bioavailability of Slow Release Formulations

The extent to which a first pass drug is sensitive to input rate should be apparent by a higher AUC after bolus doses of conventional formulations in comparison to the slow release formulation when the same dose is administered.

According to Wagner [3], AUC for zero order input with a slow release formulation can be calculated using:

$$AUC_{0-\tau(\text{zero order})} = \frac{K_m\,D_m}{(V_m - R_0)} \tag{3}$$

AUC for the dosage interval during application of a drug with conventional release characteristics is given by:

$$AUC_{0-\tau(\text{bolus})} = \frac{D_m}{V_m} (D_m/2V + C_{\text{min(ss)}} + K_m) \tag{4}$$

where D_m = bolus dose
V = volume of distribution for a one compartment model
$C_{\text{min(ss)}}$ = minimum steady state concentration when multiple oral doses are continued to steady state at intervals of τ.

(V_m (469 mg/day) and K_m (48.8 ng/ml) for propranolol were determined using the methods cited above).

The bioavailability loss using slow release preparations can thus be predicted by plotting the ratio $AUC_{0-\tau(\text{zero order})}/AUC_{0-\tau(\text{bolus})}$ (see also global equation in Appendix eq.[5]) as a function of R_0 (Fig. 3). If Michaelis-Menten kinetics were not present over the range of drug input rates being studied then the plot would be a straight line.

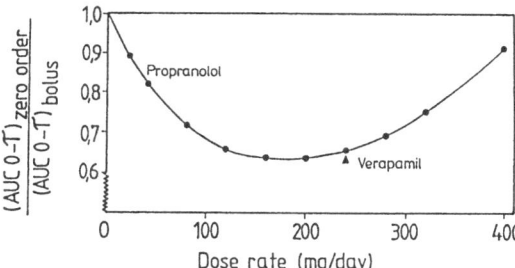

Fig. 3
The ratio of $AUC_{0-\tau(\text{zero order})}/AUC_{0-\tau(\text{bolus})}$ plotted against the drug input rate for propranolol using calculated values for V_m and K_m [3]. The single point marked with triangle is experimental data obtained under steady state conditions with slow release verapamil (Based on data [21]).

Dose — AUC Relationships

In those studies where the dose range has been large enough, as in the propranolol study of Silber et al. [13] who applied doses of 40, 80, 160, 240, and 320 mg, then a curvilinear relationship between dose and AUC is apparent and similar findings have been reported by others [14, 15].

On the other hand some investigators have reported a linear relationship between dose and AUC of propranolol [16, 17], verapamil [18] and nifedipine [19, 20]. At first sight such observations appear incompatible with the concept of Michaelis-Menten first pass metabolism. They have however been made using only a few dosage points grouped over a relatively narrow dosage range and none include dosage points corresponding to the low rates of input produced by slow release formulations which would be necessary for fully characterising the shape of the curve (Fig. 4). Furthermore, depending on the dissolution conditions in the GI-tract and differences in tablet size and surface area/mass ratio, a 10 mg tablet may produce much higher portal concentrations than a slow release formulation, but have a drug delivery rate which is not proportionally higher than a 5 mg dose.

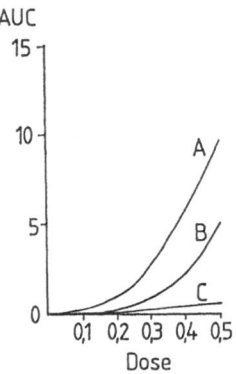

Fig. 4

Simulation showing disproportionate increase in AUC when hepatic drug metabolism is saturated after oral application. The three curves are for drugs A, B and C having different intrinsic hepatic clearance. Modified after Rowland [29].

Effect of Drug Input Rate on the First Pass Metabolism of Verapamil

Using predictions of AUC after 'bolus' doses and zero order input as shown in Fig. 3, Wagner [3] concluded that the bioavailability of verapamil is much less sensitive to input rate than propranolol. However, the sensitivity of verapamil may be higher than anticipated from these results since the estimates of V_m (575 mg/day) and K_m (133 ng/ml) used, derived by plotting Cl_{ss} versus dose rate (eg 80 mg/6h) (see appendix Eqn. 6), may have been overestimated. The reason for this is that they were based on the assumption that the intrinsic clearance of relatively high single doses of 80 mg and 120 mg in different groups of subjects, provided the actual Cl_i. If these clearances are less than the true Cl_i, then the values for K_m and V_m are higher than the true values. More suitable data for calculation of K_m and V_m of verapamil in which two or more low dose rates have been studied during steady state application in the same group of subjects does not seem to be available.

Data from the steady state study of Mantilla et al. [21] in which Isoptin SR 120 with an estimated mean zero order input rate 10 mg/h was compared with a conventional (bolus) release 80 mg tablet (Table 1) gave the calculated single point for verapamil plotted in Fig. 3. It shows that the effect of input rate on the biovailability of verapamil at the input value shown is similar in magnitude to that seen with propranolol.

Further evidence that input rate of verapamil is important was suggested by the relatively low $C_{ss(min)}$ found in 4 patients with hypertrophic obstructive cardiomyopathy who were treated with slow release verapamil (Isoptin Retard® 120) at daily doses of 600–720 mg [22].

Table 2 summarises the effect of input rate on bioavailability for slow release verapamil formulations with differing in vitro dissolution rates. The formulations investigated have been arranged according to t_{max}. Bühler et al. [23] examined 3 experimental formulations A, B and C containing 240 mg verapamil-HCl and having in vitro dissolution times (MDT = Mean dissolution time; approximately equal to time required to dissolve 60% of the total drug content) of 3.1 h, 1.8 h and 1.4 h. Formulation A with the slowest dissolution rate had the lowest AUC whereas formulation C, with the fastest dissolution rate had the highest AUC.

Rietbrock et al. [24] observed analogous results with 3 commercial preparations, Durasoptin SR 240 mg, Isoptin SR 240 mg and Veramex SR 240 mg (Table 2). The AUC

Table 1. Comparison of slow release and standard verapamil tablets at steady state

	Formulation	Dose (mg)	Subjects	t_{max} (h)	C_{max} (ng/ml)	$AUC_{0-\tau}$ (h·ng/ml)	Relative bioavail-ability	
Mantilla et al.	Isoptin-SR	120 bid		4.1	126	1075	64%	Steady state (5 days)
[21]	Orion	80 tid	Healthy (n = 12)	1.5	194	863	100%	

Table 2. Absorption characteristics of verapamil slow release (SR) formulations

Author	Formulation	Dose (mg)	Subjects	t_{max} (h)	C_{max} (ng/ml)	AUC (h·ng/ml)	Relative bioavail-ability (within study)	
Bühler et al. [23]	Isoptin SRA	240		6	49	660	56%	
	Isoptin SRB	240	Healthy (n = 18)	4	65	1064	90%	single dose median values
	Isoptin SRC	240		3	127	1182	100%	
Rietbrock et al. [24]	Durasoptin	240		17	31	628*	52%	
	Isoptin SR	240	Healthy (n = 14)	8	93	1278*	105%	single dose
	Veramex SR	240		5	111	1219*	100%	
Barbieri et al. [25]	Isoptin SR	120	Cardiac patients	5.4	35	504	65%	single dose
	Isoptin	120	(n = 6)	1.6	175	766	100%	
* AUC_{0-48h};								

of Veramex SR with the shortest t_{max} is lower than expected but this is explained by the in vitro dissolution results which showed that less than 70% of the tablets' stated content is released (Fig. 5). The release rate of Durasoptin SR was so slow that the low bioavailability may in part be due to elimination of undissolved drug in the faeces during the 2-day blood collection period (Fig. 6). The study of Barbieri et al. [25] carried out in cardiac patients having a normal cardiac index is unique in that it is the only study available so far in which equal doses of slow release and standard verapamil have been compared (Table 2). At equal dose rates, the slow release formulation has a much smaller C_{max}, and greatly reduced AUC and biovailability (-35%) with a t_{max} prolonged 4-fold.

Fig. 5

In vitro dissolution profile* of 3 commercially available slow release formulations of verapamil containing 240 mg. Paddle method; n = 6. Corresponding dissolutions-times are shown (Rietbrock et al. 1987).

	Durasoptin	Isoptin RR retard	Veramex retard
Dissolution** time (h)	>>7	4.5	1.5

* The dissolution profiles of these 3 formulations differ markedly and therefore MDT could not be used. Isoptin SR (Knoll AG) and Durosoptin (Durachemie) exhibited a constant release rate over 7h. The amount released in this interval differed markedly however, 90% and 25% (!) respectively. In the system used (Paddle method with artificial gastric/intestinal juice pH 1 − pH 7.6) Veramex (Labaz) tablets showed a first order release profile where the amount of drug released did not exceed 70% of the tablet contents.

** Estimated as the time required for the release process to be 60% complete.

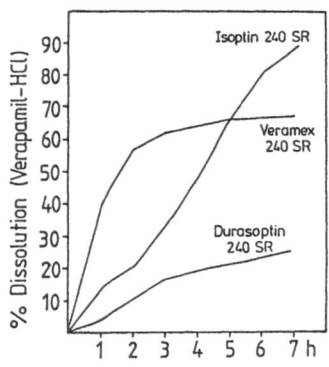

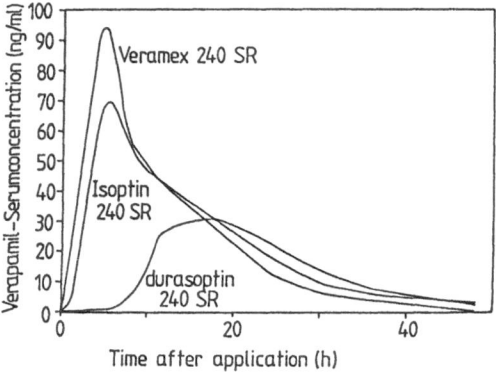

Fig. 6

Plasma concentration-time profile of verapamil following oral application of 3 commercially available 240 mg slow release formulation having widely different release characteristics.

These data show that as the in vitro dissolution rate decreases and t_{max} becomes more prolonged the bioavailability falls. Verapamil thus exhibits non-linear first pass metabolism and a considerable gain in bioavailability (at least 2-fold) can be achieved when the contents of a tablet are released rapidly.

Effect of Drug Input Rate on the First Pass Metabolism of Nifedipine

Nifedipine, like verapamil and propranolol, undergoes a first pass effect but the oral bioavailability, 40–50%, is greater. Nifedipine is a most sparingly soluble drug especially in aqueous solvents and this has lead to the use of liquid filled capsules as well as tablets and dragees for oral therapy. Nifedipine administered in capsules is absorbed immediately from the GI-tract without having to pass from the solid to the liquid phase and this is reflected in the short t_{max} (Table 3 [26]). Thus nifedipine in solid form, e.g. dragees, when compared with liquid filled capsules, appears as a 'pseudo' sustained release form. Thus the bioavailability of dragees is 30% less than that for liquid filled capsules as would be expected for drugs exhibiting Michaelis-Menten first pass metabolism.

The slow release nifedipine products Aprical SR 40 mg and 60 mg (Rentschler), based on a fatty acid alcohol matrix, are notable for their slow initial dissolution rate but near complete dissolution within 7 h (Fig. 7). The prolonged release characteristics are appropriate for a once daily application but the bioavailability is low in accord with a Michaelis-Menten kinetic (Table 4). With a dissolution rate about half that for nifedipine in Adalat SR (Bayer) the AUC of the 40 mg tablet is reduced by more than 50% with the result that

Table 3. Comparison of the absorption characteristics of nifedipine capsules and dragees

Author		Dose (mg)	Subjects	t_{max} (h)	C_{max} (ng/ml)	AUC_{tau} (h · ng/ml)	Relative bioavailability
Kees et al. [26]	Stada dragees	10	Healthy	1.40	28	119	70%
	Adalat caps	10	(n = 12)	0.54	73	171	100%

Table 4. Absorption characteristics of nifedipine slow release formulations, (Results of a steady state study over 6 days)

	Dose (mg)	Subjects	t_{max} (h)	C_{max} (ng/ml)	AUC_{0-24h} (h · ng/ml)	Relative bioavailability
Aprical SR	1 × 60		3–6	29	415	58%
Aprical SR	1 × 40	Healthy (n = 10)	–	19	210	44%
Adalat SR	20mg bid		2–3	39	477	100%
* Time for release of 60% of contents; approx. equal to MDT.						

Fig. 7.

In vitro dissolution profile of Adalat SR 20 mg tablets and Aprical SR 40 mg and 60 mg capsules. Paddle method; n = 4. Corresponding dissolution times are shown below

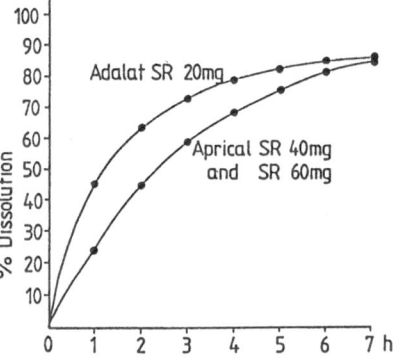

	Adalat SR 20	Aprical SR 40	Aprical SR 60
Dissolution* time (h)	1.7	3.5	3.6

* Estimated as the time required for the release process to be 60% complete.

the difference in bioavailability between Aprical 40 once daily and Adalat SR 20 mg bid determined under steady state conditions is greater than that between Isoptin SR 120 and the 120 mg conventional release dragee and between slow and conventional release propranolol. The greater bioavailability of Aprical 60 compared to Aprical 40 is not due to differences in release characteristics but is predicted from the Michaelis-Menten metabolism.

Discussion and Conclusions

The data presented must be regarded as strong evidence for the existence of Michaelis-Menten first pass metabolism not only for propranolol but also for verapamil and nifedipine. This conclusion is of considerable significance for the interpretation of bioavailability studies with these drugs.

Depending on the choice of dose and dose interval of the conventional release formulation used for comparison it is possible to obtain bioavailability data showing *superiority*, *equivalence* or *bioavailability-loss* with the slow release form. An examination of the studies of Dunn et al. [27] and Bühler et al. [28] will help to demonstrate this (Table 5).

In the single dose study of Bühler et al. [28] the 240 mg slow release formulation appears to be bioequivalent with conventional release Isoptin 120 mg because, according to Michaelis-Menten kinetics, doubling the dose reduces the difference in drug input rate between the two formulations. Similarly, in the study of Dunn et al. [27] the relative bioavailability of Verexamil appears far superior (160%) to that for verapamil solution partly or wholly because the dose disparity between slow release verapamil and solution is effectively 3:1.

The effects of a Michaelis-Menten kinetic on first pass metabolism are greater when determined under steady state conditions and thus the relative bioavailability of a slow release formulation can be overestimated in single dose studies. The relative bioavailability of Isoptin SR 120 mg in comparison with standard release tablets was 89% after single doses but only 64% after 5 days treatment [21]. This is because the effect of high steady state drug concentrations in the liver on bioavailability will be more marked at higher drug input rates.

Table 5. Absorption characteristics of verapamil slow release (SR) formulations

Bühler et al. [28]	Isoptin SR	240	Healthy (n = 7)	4	51	694	104%	Single dose median values
	Isoptin	120		1	109	334	100%	
Dunn et al. [27]	Verexamil SR	250	Healthy (n = 10)	4	156	1484	160%	"Single dose"
	Solution	3×83		1	69	923	100%	mean values

Thus, the relative bioavailability will be overestimated if:

a) Single doses are compared.
b) The dose of the slow release preparation is greater than that for the conventional release formulation.
c) The dosage interval of the conventional formulation is reduced.

Slow release formulations of cardiovascular drugs with marked first pass effects are being increasingly employed and are finding acceptance because of the benefits of reduced side effects in the early post dose period and the need for less frequent dosage. The optimisation of the clinical goals appears inherently coupled with the need to use higher daily dosages because of a Michaelis-Menten absorption kinetic. The present study has shown that the slower the dissolution rate the lower, 'ipso facto', will be the bioavailability. Slow release drugs therefore cannot be considered as inferior or as having poor quality on the basis of bioavailability alone.

A successful slow release formulation is one in which the release rate is slow enough to provide the required prolongation in t_{max} and pharmacological effect but fast enough to maintain a sufficiently high C_{max} and bioavailability.

Appendix

The loss in AUC in a slow release formulation under steady state conditions can be expressed as the quotient:

$$\frac{AUC_{0-\tau(\text{zero order})}}{AUC_{0-\tau(\text{bolus})}}$$

Assuming a one compartment model, Wagner has shown that this ratio can be expressed by the equation:

$$\frac{1}{1-r} \cdot \frac{1}{1 + D_m/V \cdot K_m \, (1/2 + \frac{1}{e^Q - 1})} \tag{5}$$

Where τ = uniform dosage interval for the bolus doses

r = Zero order input rate as a fraction of the V_m; $r = R_0/V_m$

R_0 = Zero order input rate

D_m = Maintenance dose at steady-state; $D_m = R_0 \cdot \tau$

V = volume of distribution

V_m = Pooled maximal velocity of metabolism (mass/time)

VK_m = Pooled Michaelis constant in terms of mass

Q = A dimensionless parameter that replaced $\beta\tau$ as an exponential exponent when Michaelis-Menten kinetics are operative; $Q = (1-r)\beta\tau = (V_m\tau - D_m)/VK_m = (V_m - R_0)\tau/VK_m$

β = Limiting apparent elimination rate constant. $\beta = V_m/VK_m$.

When Michaelis-Menten kinetics apply and assuming a mammillary model with central compartment elimination then:

$$Cl_{ss} = \frac{V_m - R}{K_m} \tag{6}$$

where R = Dose rate (eg. 80 mg/6 h)
and a plot of Cl_{ss} versus R will be a straight line with intercept of V_m/K_m and slope equal to $-1/K_m$ [7].

References

[1] A.G. de Boer, D.D. Breimer: Rectal absorption: Portal or systemic. In: *Drug absorption* (L.F. Prescott, W.S. Nimmo, Eds.), Adis Press, New York, p. 61–72 (1981).

[2] J. Koch-Weser, P.J. Schechter: Slow-release preparations in perspective. In: *Drug absorption* (L.F. Prescott, W.S. Nimmo, Eds.), Adis Press, New York, p. 217–227 (1981).

[3] J.G. Wagner: Propranolol: Pooled Michaelis-Menten parameters and the effect of input rate on bioavailability. *Clin. Pharm. Ther.*, 37, 481–487 (1985).

[4] D. Dvornik, M. Kraml, J. Dubuc, M. Fencik, D. Weidler, J.F. Mullane: Propranonol concentrations in healthy men given 80 mg daily in divided doses: Effect of food and circadian variation. *Curr. Ther. Res.*, 32, 214–224 (1982).

[5] D.C. Garg, R.C. Duncan, A. Mishriki, M.S. Jallad, M. Kraml, M. Fencik, D.J. Weidler: Comparative pharmacokinetics and pharmacodynamics following single and multiple doses of conventional and long-acting propranolol. *Clin. Pharm. Ther.*, 35, 242 (Abst. No. A25) (1984).

[6] K. Ohashi, A. Ebihara, K. Kondo, M. Usami: Clinical pharmacokinetics and pharmacological actions of a long-acting formulation of propranolol. *Arzneimittelforsch.*, 34, 507–512 (1984).

[7] J.W. Wagner: Predictability of verapamil steady state plasma levels from single dose data explained. *Clin. Pharm. Ther.*, 36, 1–4 (1984).

[8] M. Shomerus, B. Spiegelhalder, B. Stieren, M. Eichelbaum: Physiological disposition of verapamil in man. *Cardiovasc. Res.*, 10, 605–612 (1976).

[9] J.A. Clements, R.C. Heading, W.S. Nimmo, L.F. Prescott: Kinetics of acetominophen absorption and gastric emptying in man. *Clin. Pharm. Ther.*, 24, 420–431 (1978).

[10] O.P. Asthana, B.G. Woodcock, M. Wenchel, K.H. Frömming, L. Schwabe, N. Rietbrock: Verapamil disposition and effect on PQ-intervals after buccal, oral and intravenous administration. *Arzneim. Forschung.* 34, 498–502 (1984).

[11] B.G. Woodcock, P. Wörner, N. Rietbrock, L. Schwabe, K.H. Frömming: Pharmakokinetik und Pharmakodynamik von Verapamil bei gesunden Versuchspersonen nach einmaliger oraler und sublingualer Applikation. *Arzneim. Forschung*, 32, 1567–1571 (1982).

[12] G.R. Wilkinson: Statistical estimation in enzyme kinetics. *Biochem. J.*, 80, 324–332 (1961).

[13] B.M. Silber, N.H.G. Holford, S. Riegelman: Dose-dependent elimination of propranolol and its major metabolites in humans. *J. Pharm. Sci.*, 72, 725–732 (1983).

[14] D.G. Shand, R.E. Rango: The disposition of propranolol. 1. Elimination during oral absorption in man. *Pharmacology*, 7, 159–168 (1972).

[15] T. Walle, E.C. Convadi, K. Walle, T.C. Fagan, T.E. Gaffney: The predictable relationship between plasma levels and dose during chronic propranolol therapy. *Clin. Phar. Ther.*, 24, 668–677 (1978).

[16] L. Borgström, C.G. Johansson, H. Larsson, R. Leander: Pharmacokinetics of propranolol. *J. Pharmacokin. Biopharm.*, 9, 419–429 (1981).

[17] G.P. Mould, J. Clough, B.A. Morris, G. Stout, V. Marks: Propranolol radioimmunoassay and its use in the study of its pharmacokinetics following low doses. *Biopharm. Drug Dispos.*, 2, 49–57 (1981).

[18] R.G. McAllister, E.B. Kirsten: The pharmacology of verapamil IV. Pharmacokinetics and drug effects after single intravenous and oral doses in normal subjects. *Clin. Phar. Ther.*, 31, 418–426 (1982).

[19] O. Banzet, J.N. Cohn, M. Thibonnier, E. Singlas, J.M. Alexandre, P. Corvol: Acute antihypertensive effect and pharmacokinetics of a tablet preparation of nifedipine. *Eur. J. Clin. Pharmacol.*, 24, 145–150 (1983).

[20] K.D. Rämsch: Zur Pharmakokinetik von Nifedipin. *Schwerpunkt d. Medizin.*, 4, 55–61 (1981).

[21] J. Mattila, R. Mäntylä, J. Taskinen, P. Männisto: Pharmacokinetics of sustained release verapamil after a single administration and at steady state. *Eur. J. Drug Met. Pharmacokinet.*, 10, 133–138 (1985).

[22] B.G. Woodcock, R. Hopf, N. Rietbrock: Verapamil and norverapamil plasma concentrations during long-term therapy in patients with hypertrophic obstructive cardiomyopathy. *J. Cardiovasc. Pharmacol.*, 2, 17–23 (1980).

[23] V. Bühler, H. Einig, E. Kirsten, B. Stieren, M. Hollmann: *Verapamil pharmacokinetics with slow release formulations* (Abstract.) IUPHAR 9th International Congress of Pharmacology, London (1984a).

[24] N. Rietbrock, M. Kausch, R. Heidemann, J. Neff-Schwenger, B.G. Woodcock, G. Menke: Bioverfügbarkeit bei Retardierung von Ca-Antagonisten und Isosorbid-5-nitrat. *Therapiewoche*. In press. (1987).

[25] E. Barbieri, R. Padrini, D. Piovan, M. Toffoli, G. Cargnelli, G. Trevi, M. Ferrari: Plasma levels and urinary excretion of verapamil, norverapamil, N-dealkylverapamil (D617), N-dealkylnorverapamil (D620) following oral administration of a slow-release preparation. *Int. J. Clin. Pharm. Res.*, 2, 99–107 (1985).

[26] F. Kees, W. Dittrich, P.W. Lücker, N. Wetzelberger, H. Grobecker: Pharmakokinetik von Nifedipin. *Münchener Med., Wschr.*, 128, 15–17 (1986).

[27] J.M. Dunn, P.E. Groth: Verapamil – A once daily dosage: Pharmacokinetic and pharmacodynamic observation. *Curr. Ther. Res.*, 38, 572–578 (1985).

[28] V. Bühler, H. Einig, B. Stieren, M. Hollmann: Pharmacokinetics of verapamil sustained release formulation with multiple applications. *Naunyn Schmiedeberg's Arch. Pharmacol.*, 325, Suppl., Abs. 344 (1984b).

[29] M. Rowland: Assessment of drug absorption: Pharmacokinetic interpretation and limitations. In: *Drug absorption* (L.F. Prescott, W.S. Nimmo, Eds.), Adis Press, New York, p. 285–296 (1981).

Absorption of Caffeine in Patients with Gastric Stasis and after partial gastrectomy (Billroth II)

D. Brachtel, E. Richter

Medical Department of Krankenanstalt Mutterhaus der Borromäerinnen, D-5500 Trier; University Hospital Centre, D-8700 Würzburg

Summary

Caffeine pharmacokinetics after oral administration (tablets; 366,1 mg) were studied in patients with gastric stasis or after Billroth II partial gastrectomy. A significantly slowed absorption rate could be demonstrated in gastric stasis by mean of the lower absorption rate constant and of the prolonged peak time. The absorption rate was found to be unchanged after Billroth II partial gastrectomy. The significantly lower average of the peak concentration, of the area under the serum concentration-time curve AUC and of AUC x elimination rate constant probably reflect reduced bioavailability of caffeine in gastric stasis and after Billroth II partial gastrectomy.

Caffeine is a model compound for quantitative evaluation of liver function [1]. In healthy volunteers it is rapidly and completely absorbed [2]. As only 20% of the orally administered dose is absorbed from the stomach [3], it was examined whether an impairment of gastric emptying due to gastric stasis or Billroth II partial gastrectomy affect the absorption rate or the bioavailability of caffeine.

Methods

Patients with gastric stasis and patients who had undergone 2/3-gastrectomy (Billroth II) with normal anastomotic function were studied and compared to a control group. 5 ml blood samples were taken at 15, 30, 60, 120, 240, 480, 720 and 1440 minutes following oral administration of 366,1 mg caffeine given as compressed tablets. The serum caffeine concentration was determined by gas chromatography [4] and pharmacokinetic parameters were calculated by the computer program PEROS (ICS Comp., Frankfurt/M., FRG) on the basis of a one-compartment open model with first order absorption kinetics. Statistical analysis was carried out using the U-test according to Mann-Whitney.

Results

In patients with gastric stasis absorption of caffeine is significantly delayed and slowed (Fig. 1) compared to a control group (t_{lag} $9,9 \pm 13,8$ vs $1,8 \pm 7,8$ min, $p < 0,05$), while after 2/3-gastrectomy absorption rate is not affected (t_{lag} $0,8 \pm 1,1$ min). AUC, AUC $\times$ K_E and peak serum concentrations in gastric stasis (4874 ± 3972 mg $\times$ min/l; $8,9 \pm 3,2$ mg/l; $5,9 \pm 1,8$ µg/ml) and after partial gastrectomy (2539 ± 1180 mg $\times$ min/l; $10,1 \pm 3,7$ mg/l; $7,5 \pm 2,6$ µg/ml) were significantly reduced as compared to control data (9204 ± 6136 mg $\times$ min/l; $20,8 \pm 10,6$ mg/l; $17,7 \pm 9,4$ µ/ml) (Fig. 2). In contrast, data of clearance and volume of distribution in gastric stasis ($2,08 \pm 1,34$ ml/min/kg, $p < 0,01$; $49,9 \pm 21,3$ l, $p < 0,001$) and after Billroth II ($2,69 \pm 1,02$ ml/min/kg, $p < 0,005$; $42,3 \pm 13,4$ l, $p < 0,01$) were significantly higher as compared with the control group ($0,79 \pm 0,47$ ml/min/kg; $23,2 \pm 9,9$ l). The proportion of smokers in the group of patients with gastric stasis was twice as high [2/8] and in patients after Billroth II six times higher [4/5] as compared with the control group [2/15].

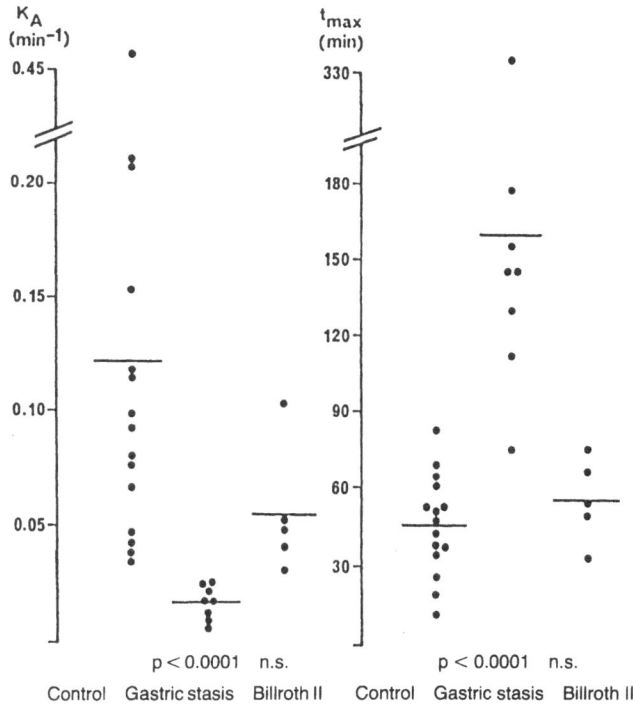

Fig. 1

Absorption rate constant (K_A) and peak time (t_{max}) after oral administration of 366,1 mg of caffeine in patients with gastric stasis and in patients with 2/3-gastrectomy (Billroth II) as compared with a control group.

109

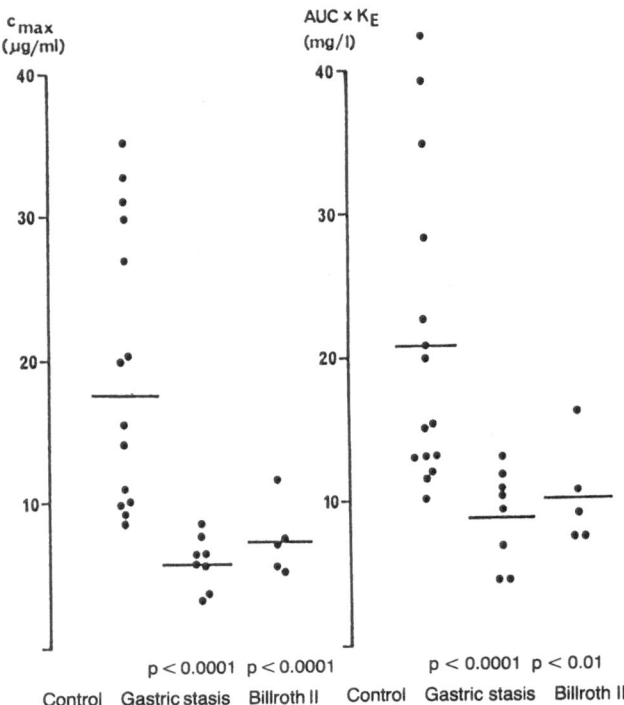

Fig. 2
Peak concentration (c_{max}), area under the serum concentration-time curve (AUC) and AUC × elimination rate constant (K_E) after oral administration of 366,1 mg of caffeine in patients with gastric stasis and in patients with 2/3-gastrectomy (Billroth II) as compared with a control group.

Discussion

Orally administered caffeine is mainly absorbed from the small intestine [2]. This explains the delayed absorption of this test substance in gastric stasis, while after partial gastrectomy (Billroth II) without grossly impaired gastric emptying the rate of caffeine absorption is not affected. Gastric emptying seems to be the rate limiting step of caffeine absorption – which is comparable to the mechanisms of paracetamol absorption [5]. Significantly lower values of peak concentration, AUC and AUC × K_E probably reflect decreased bioavailability of caffeine in gastric stasis and after Billroth II and thus may influence the assessment of caffeine clearance.

References

[1] E. Renner, A. Wietholtz, P. Huguenin, M. Arnaud, R. Preisig: Caffeine: a model compound for measuring liver function. *Hepatology* 4, 38–46 (1984).

[2] J. Blanchard, S.J.A. Sawers: The absolute bioavailability of caffeine in man. *Eur. J. Clin. Pharmacol.* 24, 93–98 (1983).

[3] T.E. Chvasta, A.R. Cooke: Emptying and absorption of caffeine from the human stomach. *Gastroenterology* 61, 838–843 (1971).

[4] H. Heusler, E. Richter: Quantitative Bestimmung von Coffein in biologischen Flüssigkeiten mit Hilfe der Gaschromatographie und N-selektiven Detektion. In: N. Rietbrock, B.G. Woodcock, A.H. Straib, eds. *Theophylline and other Methylxantines.* Vieweg Braunschweig-Wiesbaden, 291–298 (1982).

[5] J.A. Clements, R.C. Heading, W.S. Nimmo, L.F. Prescott: Kinetics of acetaminophen absorption and gastric emptying in man. *Clin. Pharmacol. Ther.* 24, 420–431 (1978).

Kurzfassung der round-table-Diskussion

D. Loew und A.H. Staib

Folgende Schwerpunkte wurden erörtert:

1. Übertragbarkeit der mit den vorgestellten Methoden gewonnenen pharmakokinetischen Daten auf klinische Bedingungen. Hinweis z.b. auf die unter Endoskopie auftretenden lokalen Irritationen, auf die Freisetzung vasoaktiver Mediatoren und deren Wirkungen auf den Resorptionsprozeß.
2. Lokale Konzentrationsabhängigkeit der Absorptionskonstanten, Beispiel Digoxin, Interaktion z.B. mit Antibiotika.
3. Problem der Lokalisationsgenauigkeit und Strahlenbelstung bei HF-Kapseluntersuchungen.
4. Differenzierung Darminhalt-bedingter, Darmwand-abhängiger (Metabolisierung) und anderer Ursachen mit Einfluß auf die Bioverfügbarkeit.
5. Übertragbarkeit der hier vorgestellten Absorptionsstudien auf die Entwicklung von Retardpräparaten.

ad. 1:

Frage
Inwieweit sind die aus Absorptionsstudien gewonnenen pharmakokinetischen Daten von klinisch-therapeutischer Bedeutung, speziell wenn sie unter endoskopischen Bedingungen gewonnen wurden? Jeder, der eine Endoskopie durchführt, weiß, daß vor der Endoskopie Substanzen benutzt werden, die eine gewisse lokale Hyperämie verursachen und weiterhin, daß die verschiedenen Endoskopie-Formen (z.B. Gastroskopie oder Coloskopie) unangenehme Untersuchungsverfahren sind, den Patienten mit Schmerzen belasten, wodurch u.a. vasoaktive Substanzen, Katecholamine und lokal Prostaglandine freigesetzt werden. Hierdurch werden doch mit hoher Wahrscheinlichkeit die gemessenen pharmakokinetischen Parameter beeinflußt.

Antwort
Wir wissen, daß bei derartigen Untersuchungen keine physiologischen Bedingungen vorliegen. Durch einen erfahrenen Endoskopiker lassen sich negative Einflüsse weitgehend reduzieren. Über die Freisetzung von vasoaktiven Substanzen, Katecholamine und Prostaglandine liegen bisher keine Ergebnisse vor.
Hinweis aus dem Auditorium: Der hier angesprochene Gesichtspunkt bedarf einer weiteren Vertiefung.

Hinweis aus dem Auditorium:
Nach Verabreichung von Piretanid als Tabletten oder als Lösung werden variable Bioverfügbarkeitswerte beobachtet. Nach Verabreichung von Piretanid im Magen wurden aber gleiche Plasmaspiegelverläufe wie nach normaler oraler Applikation gefunden. Nach Verabreichung von Piretanid in das Duodenum wurden weiterhin bereits nach 10 Minuten Spitzenkonzentrationen erreicht. Hieraus kann geschlossen werden, daß die verschiedenen Untersuchungstechniken keinen Einfluß auf die Absorption hatten.

ad. 2:

Diskussionsbemerkung

Untersuchungen aus den 70er Jahren über die Absorption des Digoxins aus dem Colon zeigten, daß eine Absorption der Substanz erfolgt. Bei gleichzeitiger Verabreichung von Antibiotika konnten erhöhte Digoxinkonzentrationen und eine entsprechend erhöhte Bioverfügbarkeit nachgewiesen werden. Der Mechanismus ist unklar. Die Resultate zeigen aber, daß bei entsprechender Comedikation, besonders bei Substanzen mit einer geringen therapeutischen Breite, Probleme resultieren können.

Frage

Wie können derartige Interaktionseffekte untersucht und interpretiert werden?

Antwort

Es gibt Untersuchungen über die Digoxin-Absorption an der Ratte von Rietbrock, die später von anderen Untersuchern bestätigt wurden. Die Resultate zeigen, daß die Absorptionskonstante des Digoxins von der augenblicklich herrschenden Konzentration abhängig ist, d.h., daß bei hoher Konzentration eine hohe Absorptionskonstante und bei niedriger eine entsprechend geringere Absorptionskonstante gefunden wird.

Gleiches wurde später von Anderson für den Menschen nachgewiesen. Eine Erklärung bietet sich nach Lauterbach dadurch an, daß parallel Absorptions- und Sekretionsprozesse ablaufen. Durch Einstellung eines Gleichgewichtes entsteht so der Eindruck, daß die Substanzen zuerst bolusartig absorbiert und später, obwohl lokal noch ein genügendes Substanzangebot angenommen werden muß, überhaupt keine Absorption mehr stattfindet.

ad. 3:

Frage

Wie sicher ist die Lokalisation der HF-Kapsel im Gastrointestinaltrakt möglich?

Antwort

Bei der röntgenologischen Lokalistion ergeben sich gelegentlich tatsächlich Probleme. Der erfahrene Röntgenologe kann jedoch bestimmte Lokalisationen eindeutig definieren. In unseren Untersuchungen (Demonstration von entsprechenden Röntgenaufnahmen) konnten wir bestätigen, daß vom Magen bis zur Treitz'schen Falte keine Probleme auftauchen. Ferner werden im distalen Ileum und im gesamten Colonbereich in aller Regel die Lokalisationsmöglichkeiten optimal sein. Schwierigkeiten bestanden jedoch eindeutig bei der Lokalisation im Jejunum und im mittleren Ileumbereich. Es ist ferner darauf hinzuweisen, daß unter Röntgenkontrolle und anhand einer Aufnahme exakt festgestellt werden kann, ob die Kapsel geöffnet ist oder sich aus irgendwelchen Gründen vorher die Position des Öffnungsmechanismus (Nadel) verändert hat. Ferner ist festzustellen, daß eine Absorption bei den Kapseluntersuchungen immer nur distal von der Sprengungslokalisation erfolgt. Die Möglichkeit, eine Lokalisation zu präzisieren, indem Kontrastmittel gegeben wird, kann nur mit anderen Problemen (Adsorption von Wirkstoff) erkauft werden. Deshalb haben wir im allgemeinen auf diese Methode verzichtet.

Frage

Wie hoch ist die Strahlenbelastung bei der Lokalisation der HF-Kapsel?

Antwort
Unter Verwendung der bei uns erfolgten Routinetechnik ergab sich bei der Kalkulation nach 5 Durchgängen pro Person, das ist eine Versuchsrunde mit 5 Lokalisationen, etwa eine Verdoppelung der Grundbelastung durch natürliche Strahlenquellen pro Jahr. Wir halten diesen Zuwachs an Strahlenbelastung für vertretbar.

ad. 4:
Frage
Wie kann die Beeinflussung der Absorption durch die Veränderung des Darminhalts, z.B. durch Darmbakterien oder durch bestimmte Nahrungsmittelbestandteile, differenziert werden?

Antwort
Diese Einflüsse entsprechen den Bedingungen, wie sie bei normalen Bioverfügbarkeitsuntersuchungen auftreten und wie sie auch durch Berücksichtigung der first-pass-Effekte (unterschiedliche Metabolisierungsraten) ermittelt werden können. Der Hinweis, daß die Messung der Metaboliten einen Anhaltspunkt für diese Einflüsse gibt, gilt auch für bereits im Darmlumen stattfindende Metabolisierungsprozesse.

ad. 5:
Frage
Die Bedingungen der Untersuchungen, wie sie hier vorgestellt werden, stellen eine Sondersituation dar, worauf oben bereits hingewiesen wurde. Die Gefahr besteht, daß die gewonnenen Ergebnisse für die Entwicklung von Retardpräparationen überinterpretiert werden. Wie können derartige Fehler bei Interpretation von Ergebnissen ausgeschlossen werden?

Antwort
Untersuchungen wie die vorgestellten, stellen nur einen Schritt auf dem Wege zur Entwicklung einer optimalen galenischen Darreichungsform dar. Eine letzte Entscheidung ist immer nur durch Untersuchungen am Patienten möglich. Es erscheint aber wichtig, zukünftig durch diese Untersuchungen eine Richtung für einzuschlagende Methoden festzulegen. Weiterhin muß darauf hingewiesen werden, daß der Umfang von steady-state-Untersuchungen erweitert werden sollte, besonders gilt das bei Substanzen mit langen Halbwertszeiten, weniger für Retardpräparate mit unterschiedlich verzögerter Freisetzungsrate.

Zusammenfassung der Diskussionsergebnisse:

1. Methoden-bedingte Einflüsse müssen bei Absorptionsuntersuchungen berücksichtigt werden, können aber durch geeignete Versuchsplanung und durch erfahrene Untersucher auf ein Minimum reduziert werden.
2. Das Beispiel Digoxin zeigt, daß überraschende oder unerwartete Ergebnisse von Absorptionsstudien nur durch substanzspezifische und Detail-bezogene Berücksichtigung aller Faktoren interpretiert werden können.
3. Lokalisationsprobleme mit der HF-Kapsel bestehen nur im mittleren Dünndarmbereich. Die Strahlenbelastung ist kalkulierbar, sie besteht z.B. bei 5 Untersuchungsdurchgängen für einen Probanden in einer Verdoppelung der jährlichen natürlichen Strahlenbelastung.

4. Unterschiedliche Einflußursachen auf die Ergebnisse von Absorptionsstudien können auch durch Erfassung der Metaboliten-Konzentration präzisiert werden.
5. Der derzeitige technische Stand der Untersuchungsmethoden erlaubt in Hinsicht auf die Entwicklung von Retardpräparaten folgendes:
   1. Ausschluß von Resorptionsfenstern,
   2. quantitative Differenzierung zwischen verschiedenen Darmabschnitten,
   3. qualitative Differenzierung begleitender Vorgänge wie z.B. intestinaler first-pass-Effekt.

Schlußwort

A.H. Staib

Der Workshop hat die mit verschiedenen Untersuchungsmethoden erzielten Ergebnisse vergleichend dargestellt. Wir haben durch die Möglichkeit einer Diskussion von Resultaten und ein Einbringen auch außerhalb dieser Untersuchungen vorhandener Erfahrungen viel dazulernen können.

Wir konnten feststellen, daß von verschiedenen Ansatzpunkten her sehr genaue Untersuchungen der intestinalen Absorptionsvorgänge möglich sind und die technischen Voraussetzungen in den letzten Jahren eine erhebliche Verbesserung erfahren haben. Es gilt jetzt, diese Möglichkeiten für die Entwicklung in der pharmazeutischen Industrie, aber auch für die Grundlagenforschung systematisch und gezielt nutzbar zu machen. In unserem Workshop wurde dazu ein erster Ansatz gefunden.

Ich danke allen Beteiligten für die Teilnahme und ihre aktive und anregende Diskussion. Nicht zuletzt möchte ich an dieser Stelle auch den Mitarbeitern der Abteilung für ihren aktiven Einsatz bei der Vorbereitung des Workshops danken.

Ich hoffe, daß durch eine rasche Drucklegung die Resultate des Workshops einem größeren Kreis zugänglich gemacht werden können.

Dem Vieweg-Verlag danke ich für die Bereitschaft, auch diesmal Vorträge und Diskussionen der nunmehr 7. internationalen Veranstaltung unserer Abteilung für den Druck vorzubereiten und die Publikation zu ermöglichen.

Sachwortverzeichnis / Subject Index

für deutschsprachige Beiträge

For English contributions